MW01595382

From the Bedside to the HMO
A Doctor's Journey

by

Robert Whiting MD

To Dee, I hope you enjoy the book.

Bob Whiting

iUniverse, Inc.
New York   Bloomington

From the Bedside to the HMO
A Doctor's Journey

iUniverse books may be ordered through booksellers or by contacting:

iUniverse
1663 Liberty Drive
Bloomington, IN 47403
www.iuniverse.com
1-800-Authors (1-800-288-4677)

Because of the dynamic nature of the Internet, any Web addresses or links contained in this book may have changed since publication and may no longer be valid.

ISBN: 978-1-4401-2377-1 (pbk)
ISBN: 978-1-4401-2378-8 (cloth)
ISBN: 978-1-4401-2379-5 (ebk)

Printed in the United States of America

iUniverse rev. date: 3/9/2009

DEDICATION

This book is dedicated to my wife Marlene, and to our three children Lois, Marc, and Craig, for their understanding and patience in sharing their "growing up period" with all the needs of others in a small town medical practice.

ACKNOWLEDGEMENTS

It takes more than a writer, especially a newcomer, to get a book ready for publication. I have several people to thank for their help in this endeavor. First to Gerald Pattyn, for all his computer magic in sizing, formatting, and putting all the pictures in the right places. There were a few incidents in some of the chapters that were a little fuzzy in my mind, but with the help of one of our long tenured nurses, Lorraine Kuntz, her "steel trap" memory helped clear those up. Glennine Schoen, our previous office manager, helped me by proofreading and finding those little errors that creep into the text. Laurie Nelson edited the book and helped make it a bit more readable. Finally, to Dr. Elwyn Simons, who told me the interesting story about how his father "almost" discovered penicillin. Our life long association, while growing up, helped steer me in the direction of science and medicine, which eventually led me to write this book.

Contents

INTRODUCTION

There are probably as many reasons for one to write a book about one's life experiences as there are grains of sand on the beach. When I decided to start this undertaking, I had to ask myself, "What do I have to tell that makes this task worthwhile?"

I suppose that every physician throughout history believed that theirs was the age when the most significant achievements occurred. At the start of the nineteenth century, physicians had no knowledge of the tiny microorganisms called germs or "beasties," as the first microscopist, Anton von Leeuwenhoek, called them. Who knew then that they were the cause of the horrible infections that ravaged the patients following surgery and took many of their lives.

Anesthesia was not known at that time, and surgery had to be done quickly with laudanum and whiskey as the only way to relieve some of the pain of the knife. In 1846, a dentist named William Morton first demonstrated the wonderful effect of ether. Overnight, the world of painless surgery was first visited on the profession of medicine. Suddenly, surgeons were free from hearing the screams of their patients as they plied their trade in a more complete and careful manner.

Then, on the heels of this fabulous step forward, several other giants in their profession brought forth advancements and innovations for the good of all. Ignac Semmelweis, Louis Pasteur, Joseph Lister, and Robert Koch taught us how to prevent the surgical infections, and they gave us insight into the causes of other illnesses that were killing their patients. Surely, this had to be the age when all there was to know was known. This had to be the best time to be a doctor, when one could really do something positive in helping patients to recover from their afflictions.

Then, in the early 1930s, a German chemist named Gerhard Domagt was working with analine dyes, and he discovered that they had an antibacterial effect on various bacteria. His drug, called Prontosil, cured several infections, but was really brought to notoriety by a chance occurrence. He had given some of the tablets to a Baltimore physician, Dr. Perin Long, who had a child in Boston who was dying from a streptococcal infection, and he used them to save the patient. The parents were Eleanor and Franklin Roosevelt. And thus were born the sulfa drugs. It was learned later that the analine dye was split apart during digestion, and the active sulfa molecule was then released in the body to do its miracle work. In 1928, a bacteriologist, Alexander Fleming, was working at St. Mary's hospital in London, and he noted that around an old culture plate that had been exposed to the air, some colonies of mold were growing that had contaminated the plate from the air. Other bacterial contaminants were also present, but they would not grow next to to this mold. Another miracle and penicillin made its presence known, although it took over ten more years before the world was to realize its true significance. Surely, this had to be the best time to be a physician. Now we really had the magic bullet to cure the dreaded infections that were killing our patients.

When I started medical school in 1953, all of these advances were in common use. We now had, in addition to penicillin and sulfa, other drugs such as streptomycin, chloramphenacol, and tetracycline. Anesthesia had made great strides with the advent of divinyl ether, meperidine, cyclopropane, sodium pentathol, and muscle relaxants. There were very few drugs for hypertension, fluid retention, and other cardiac treatments. However, those that we could use had terrible side effects. We had yet to see all the wonderful advances in immunizations, monitors, defibrillators, laparoscopes, gastroscopes, and all the other myriads of technological advances that we now take for granted.

But, this has been my world, and I have seen both the old and the new. I have seen the beginning of Medicare, Medicaid, the phasing out of charity care, and the astronomical rise in malpractice insurance costs. Regulations, diagnosis codes, and length of hospital stays are now determined by insurance companies and the government. Mandated outpatient surgery is now dictated by the insurance companies. These changes have all come to pass during my lifetime in medicine. I think that my fifty years in medicine has seen a significant amount of new direction, and deserves some comment from someone who has seen it develop over the last half century.

Sometime the smallest of events have a profound effect in shaping our lives in a totally different direction than we would otherwise have planned. I had not really planned on medicine as a career, and it was one of those small quirks of fate that turned me from law or engineering into the profession of medicine. And so the story begins...............

CHAPTER 1
THE ENCOUNTER

It was a beautiful spring day with the sun shining in the blue sky and the temperature validating that spring was here to stay. That was the day that changed the rest of my life. It is strange how some small insignificant event can irrevocably and forever change the direction that will shape the rest of one's life. That was what happened to me on that day after school in the spring of 1949.

School had just let out and I was a little late getting out to catch the bus home, so I decided to hitchhike a ride down Westheimer street for the five miles to my home. That was when I met Elmer Schulze. I had been wondering what kind of a job that I should try to get for the summer when Elmer picked me up. It turned out that he was looking for someone to work in his small medical laboratory, washing test tubes and glassware, and generally cleaning up at the end of the day. Since no one in my family had previously been involved in anything related to medicine, I was not really thinking about that as a career. In fact, I had taken a series of very involved aptitude tests that said that I would be better satisfied with a career in law or something related to music. So much for aptitude tests! I was really planning something in science, since the desire for knowledge of nature had been awakened in me quite early when I first met my long time friend, Dr. Elwyn Simons, currently head of the Primate Center at Duke University. We met when we were ages seven and six respectively. He taught me about bugs, butterflies and dinosaurs which kept me always wanting to know more about everything. But, I am digressing.

Elmer had just left the Navy, having been a corpsman and laboratory technician. He had opened his laboratory in a medical clinic housing about six other doctors. There were three internists and three obstetricians and business was picking up. He also did the lab work for several other doctors and small clinics, and provided pickup service for the blood and specimens each day. Besides the cleanup, he needed someone to drive around town and make the pickups. All of Elmer's brothers were doctors, but he failed to make the grade in medical school, being more interested in playing jazz piano than hitting the books. Music created a bond between us when a band that I had formed started to play for school dances and dance club events held at the local country clubs. I needed a piano player that I could count on regularly. He offered me the lab job, and I invited him home to meet my parents. He arrived and noted that we had a grand piano in the home. He sat down and gave us quite a performance. I got out my saxophone and we played a few tunes together. He began to show me how to improvise by using chord progressions and rhythm variations to change up the basic melody. We really hit it off.

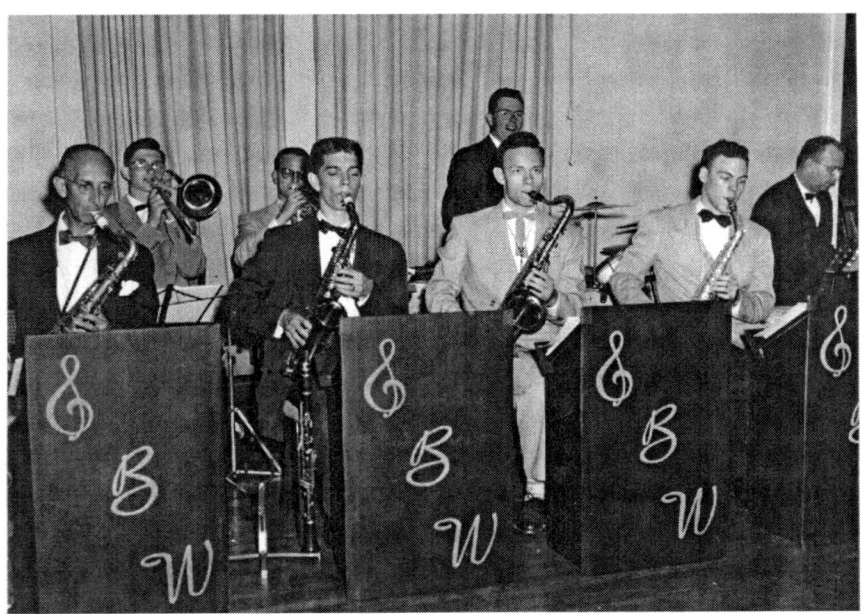

The Sparklers, my first dance band.

I started to work at the lab after school and then full time when school was out. I made the pickups, washed the glassware, and before long, he began to show me how to do a blood count, use the microscope, look at blood smears, and then to test urine. In those days we didn't have the test strips that run all of the tests with one dip of the strip. Each test had to be run separately, although we could batch a half dozen or so at one time. Urine sugars had to be tested by adding 5 drops of urine to 5 c.c. of Benedict's solution, and then boiling to develop a color change. To test for protein, one would add urine to sulfosalicylic acid, and if protein was present, it would precipitate as a cloud. I won't bore you with all of the other tests, but it was a lot more time consuming than the way we do it today. And all for only fifty cents for a complete urinalysis! Before long, I was learning to perform a venipuncture and draw blood. I got quite good at that and sometimes, when the doctors couldn't find a vein, they would send the patients down the hall to the high school student to get the blood.

Today, all test tubes are discarded, but at that time we washed out the blood, soaked them in detergent, rinsed and dried them, and used them until they were broken or so scratched that they were unusable. Likewise, all of the needles were reused after cleaning them and checking the points under the microscope to make sure that there were no barbs or blunt points. The needles were boiled, and then soaked in alcohol because we didn't have an autoclave in those days. There was never a worry about transmitting hepatitis at that time, and all of the other exotic illnesses either were not around or recognized.

After a year of working in the lab after school, I decided to change my major from chemical engineering to premed. I had been accepted by Rice University in early 1950, but was able to switch my major, since all of the first year college courses were the same for the two sciences.

Elmer had quite an influence on the direction of my life, both in directing me toward medicine and also in the musical field. He had some really great jazz musicians that would come to his house, and I would listen and try to play some of their styles. Music and the lab were able to put me through college and medical school with very little help from my parents, except for the important fact that I was able

3

to live at home during that time and have those needs provided by them.

I was never able to pursue any formal musical training outside of the school band and orchestra; however, after an initial nine months of saxophone lessons I taught myself to play the clarinet and later, the guitar. I kept the band going on weekends throughout medical school with myself on sax, Elmer on piano, Mac Cauldwell on drums, and a stand up bass player named Sam Luce, who was in my medical school class. Sam was quite an interesting fellow that also had an influence on my life, but that will be for later chapters.

As I progressed through college, several of the courses that I took helped in the lab. We had to do a lot of parasitology, including malaria slides and stool exams in the lab, and my training on site was pretty minimal. After taking the college parasitology course and completing the periodic competency tests that the state lab sends out, I got one of the highest grades for our lab evaluation. During medical school, the bacteriology and biochemistry took on added meaning since it had practical value for me which would serve me well when I opened my rural practice several years later.

CHAPTER 2
EARLY YEARS

Over the years I have heard friends and classmates say that high school was the worst time of their lives and that they would never want to relive that time again. That wasn't my experience. My parents never pushed me unduly to excel but it was somehow implied that I had to study hard until I learned everything that was presented. I certainly did not have a photographic memory, and it took a lot of work to remember most of what was taught. I did learn to read earlier and better than most children, and studying was fun and not work. There was so much to know in this world, and I set about this early in the quest for knowledge. I am sure that my first real friend and playmate, Elwyn Simons, had a lot to do with that desire.

Our acquaintance began shortly after we moved to our new home on Dryden Road in Houston. He lived half way up the block, and as soon as we had settled in he was at our door to ask if I could come out and play. Elwyn's father was a professor at Rice University (Rice Institute in those days) and his family was much more intellectually driven than my parents, who were just high school graduates and more of a typical family of the times. Elwyn and I collected butterfly specimens, watched caterpillars spin cocoons and emerge as beautiful specimens. We watched tadpoles change from eggs to wigglers and then sprout legs and develop into frogs. There were so many marvels of nature about which to learn. We read about dinosaurs, the geologic eras with their fossils, and about the evolutionary process.

Elwyn told me an interesting story regarding his father that relates to the story that I told you earlier about the discovery of penicillin by Fleming.

When Vern, Elwyn's father, was in college at Kansas University in the 1920s, he got a job in the summer with the Kansas Water Board. His job was to drive around and collect water samples from private wells to see that the water was safe to drink. He would then put a few drops of the water on agar petri dishes, incubate them and see what they grew. More than once Vern noted that a particular mold would start to grow, and that near the mold no bacteria would grow. He was told by his superiors that it was penicillium. No correlation was made of the possible implications by Vern or the Water Board people about its potential value in treating infections. This was four or five years before Fleming made the same discovery. Vern said that he almost discovered Penicillin!

High school was a fun time and I enjoyed all my teachers. Since I studied hard and made good grades, I probably received a little extra encouragement to excel. I was in a lot of extracurricular activities, including ROTC, band, orchestra, and several sports including softball, which was my forte. I applied to Rice University, and was accepted after an interview and grade average without the usual pretesting applications. SAT testing and scoring now used by college entrance boards had yet to be developed. I graduated number three in my class of four hundred and fifty and was off to college with great anticipation of an interesting future.

Rice was a tough school academically. We really had to study until late at night in order to get all the information "digested." We had great professors, but I remember one in particular, Dr. Davies, who taught biology. His teeth didn't fit right, and they were always clacking when he lectured. He was very animated, however, and kept our attention. We practically had to memorize his lectures because the tests were very predictable. If we did, we had no trouble answering the questions. Not so, with the inorganic chemistry professor. We would study all the old tests, and would feel that we were really well prepared. When the tests were passed out, our balloons were deflated, and a new wrinkle in the problem was added. There was always an extra credit question and we were graded on the curve. I would study the first question, find it impossible, and move on to the next, and then the next, feeling totally overwhelmed. The only solace was that everyone was in the same boat.

The labs were fun, but were a lot of work burning things in our ceramic crucibles, weighing substances, titrating acids out to the fourth decimal place, and reacting acids and bases to produce esters and stable salts. A few of my friends thought they would shortcut some of the work by buying titrated hydrochloric acid from Curtain Chemical company to use in the reactions instead of titrating it for themselves. Fortunately, I stuck with making my own titration and calculation. Curtain's chemist was off a few hundredths and since all of these students were using the same solution and got the same wrong answer, the lab instructor smelled a rat and penalized them accordingly.

In embryology lab we had to prepare the chicken embryos at different stages of development. We would run them through a series of dilute ethyl alcohol solutions, finally ending up with 90% concentration. At that point we would mount them on the slides. Several of us noted that on our lab counters were a number of glass stoppered bottles filled with drinkable alcohol in various concentrations, and there were no checks and balances of how much we used in our preparations. We would take a little from each bottle, being careful that no discrepancies would be obvious, and then make "purple passion punch" at our fraternity parties. There is no end to what college kids will do to obtain alcohol.

The Korean War was in progress, and being drafted was a concern since I didn't want to interrupt my education. I joined the Naval ROTC at Rice, and was therefore exempted from the draft. I would be required to sign a contract for a commission as an ensign on beginning my third year. ROTC was really interesting and did require as much study as math, chemistry, and biology, since there was a test every day on the previous day's material. I took a heavy load of all the required courses for medical school in the hope that I would be accepted after three years of college, provided that my grades were high enough. There wasn't much time for anything except classes, afternoon labs, and night time study. I did continue with my four piece dance band for some extra income, playing several times a month. I still worked at Schulze's medical lab several hours a week and full time during the summer. These part time jobs paid my tuition and still gave me a little spending money. Living at home also made it easier to cut costs.

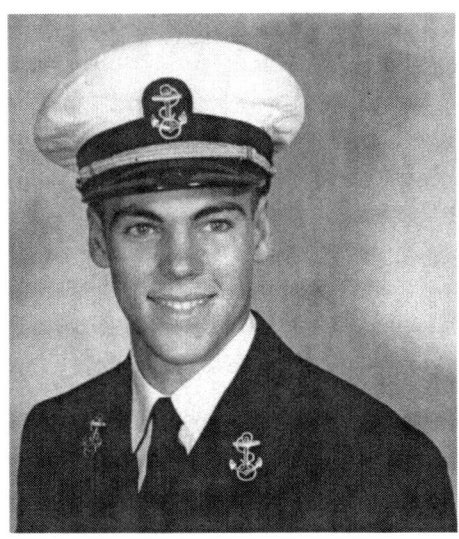

1951 ROTC Photo

I dropped Naval ROTC after the first two years and was accepted by Baylor Medical School after completing my third year of college. That kept me out of the draft until after I completed medical school. At that point, I did my military obligation in the Indian Health Service following my internship. I made many long lasting friendships in college. Several of my premed classmates were also accepted by Baylor and we entered that phase of our lives with a sense of awe and anticipation.

CHAPTER 3
SPORTS

Sports have always been a big part of my life. When I was quite young my father spent time helping me to develop coordination and sports skills. He was a member of the 1937-1938 Houston YMCA championship volleyball team that won the national championship. There was no Olympic volleyball in those days, but that would have been akin to winning the gold medal. We played various sports in the neighborhood, so we were all physically active, and no one was overweight on our block. I also would go to the "Y" when Dad played recreational volleyball in later years, and I could occasionally be the sixth man on his team if they were short a player. Since the high school volleyball coach had no interest in volleyball and was really the basketball coach, he let me be the player coach. I was able to pass on what I had learned from my father about the teamwork of setting the ball for the spiker, forming a blocking wall, and serving a floater serve. We actually did all right, and in my senior year we came in second in the Houston High School league.

However, softball was really the sport to which I gave the most attention. Dad and I would go out to Buffalo Stadium and watch the women's fastpitch games, and also the men's major city league. They had four teams in that league that competed all over the country. They had some of the best players anywhere. I used to marvel at Julian Kujawa's rise ball at close to 100 mph (or so they said) clocking it with a stopwatch. There was no little league baseball in the 1940s, but church league and city league softball was very popular. I loved to pitch, so I began to work on pitching mechanics. There were no manuals or books available to teach the fundamentals of pitching, but my father and I would watch the good pitchers in the major city league, and I would try to copy their style. Dad had pitched some amateur baseball in his younger years, and he used his pitching skills to help me develop spin on the ball. I wish that I had known then what I know now since I started coaching. After studying the excellent manuals and coaching videos that are available to develop young pitchers, I have picked up many informative tips that would have been nice to put to use fifty years ago. In those days, one just watched the better pitchers and tried to mimic their style. Maybe the term "too late, too smart" applies.

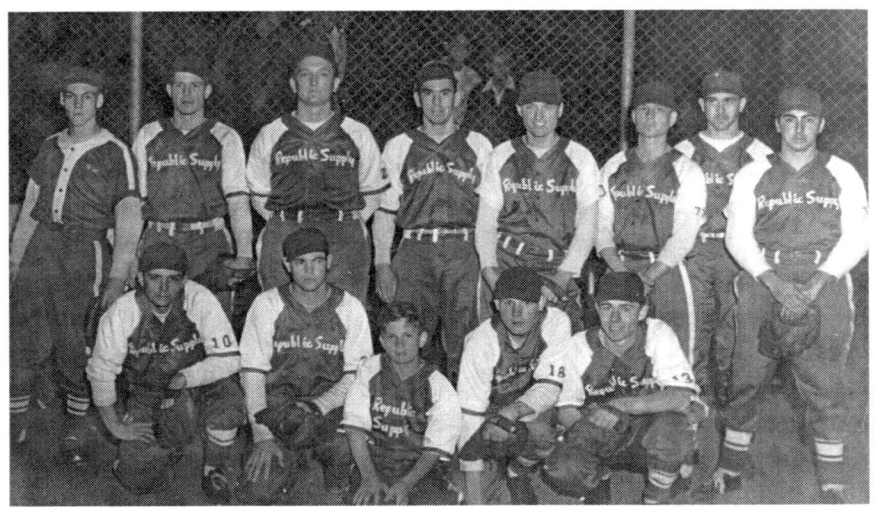

My first team at age 16.

By the time I was sixteen, I was playing in the Metropolitan league, which was one step down from the major city league. By that time I had my pitching speed up to about 70 mph, and my rise ball became my best pitch. Getting lots of underspin on the ball and watching it climb up over the spot where the batter was swinging was a great feeling. I never really concentrated much on a change-up, and just threw the rise and the drop. I had a fair curve but I didn't throw it much since the curve comes in level and is easier to hit. I managed to pitch quite a few no hit games, with three in a row my longest string.

I had always wanted to pitch against Julian Kujawa's team, but the closest I got was in 1953 when I was playing in the annual Houston

Chronicle fastpitch tournament. My team got to the quarter finals and would have met his team in the next round, but we were put out. By that time I was starting college and aside from intramural softball, there wasn't time to pitch competitively. Then it was medical school, and sports had to take a back seat. During internship, my two years in the USPHS Indian Service, and my residency, I didn't pitch. I began again in 1962 when we organized an active fastpitch league in Hardin, and we actually won the state championship once with an all star team from our league. My rise ball still had a lot of jump on it, and I got a lot of strikeouts with that pitch. When I was coaching the Hardin girls fastpitch in later years, one of the umpires called me aside and said, "I remember playing against you twenty-five years ago, and I never want to see your rise ball again."

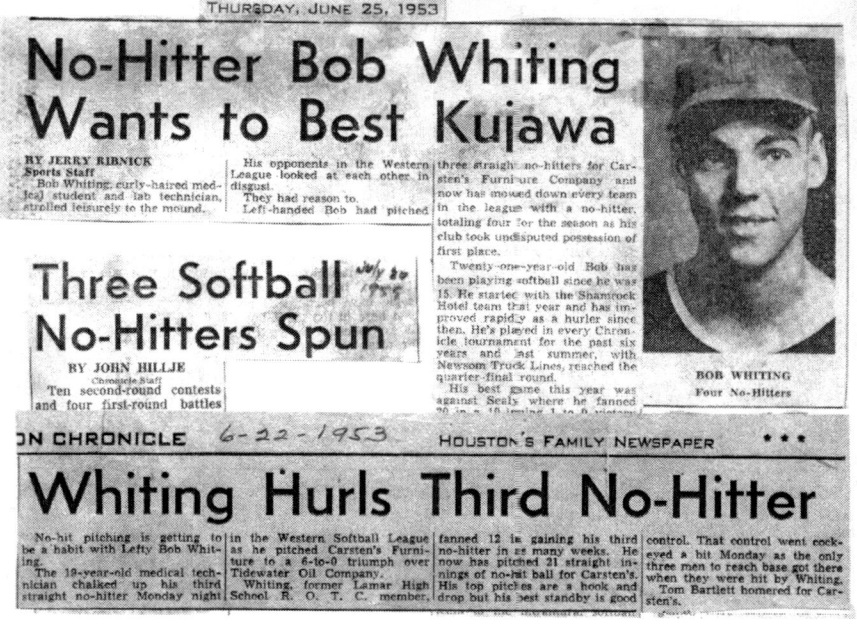

THURSDAY, JUNE 25, 1953

No-Hitter Bob Whiting Wants to Best Kujawa

BY JERRY RIBNICK
Sports Staff

Bob Whiting, curly-haired medical student and lab technician, strolled leisurely to the mound.

His opponents in the Western League looked at each other in disgust.

They had reason to.

Left-handed Bob had pitched

three straight no-hitters for Carsten's Furniture Company and now has mowed down every team in the league with a no-hitter, totaling four for the season as his club took undisputed possession of first place.

Twenty-one-year-old Bob has been playing softball since he was 15. He started with the Shamrock Hotel team that year and has improved rapidly as a hurler since then. He's played in every Chronicle tournament for the past six years and last summer, with Newsom Truck Lines, reached the quarter-final round.

His best game this year was against Sealy where he fanned

BOB WHITING
Four No-Hitters

Three Softball No-Hitters Spun

BY JOHN HILLJE
Chronicle Staff

Ten second-round contests and four first-round battles

ON CHRONICLE 6-22-1953 HOUSTON'S FAMILY NEWSPAPER • • •

Whiting Hurls Third No-Hitter

No-hit pitching is getting to be a habit with Lefty Bob Whiting.

The 19-year-old medical technician chalked up his third straight no-hitter Monday night

in the Western Softball League as he pitched Carsten's Furniture to a 6-to-0 triumph over Tidewater Oil Company.

Whiting, former Lamar High School R. O. T. C. member,

fanned 12 is gaining his third no-hitter in as many weeks. He now has pitched 21 straight innings of no-hit ball for Carsten's. His top pitches are a hook and drop but his best standby is good

control. That control went cockeyed a bit Monday as the only three men to reach base got there when they were hit by Whiting.

Tom Bartlett homered for Carsten's.

Newspaper clippings of some of my no hitter games.

There are three games in all of those years that I especially remember, and none was a no hitter. When I was fifteen and just learning to pitch, I was in a game in which I had the bases loaded and a count of three balls and no strikes on a batter with only one out. My next pitch was so wild that it hit the bat that the batter still had on his shoulder and the ball popped out in fair territory about half way between home and the pitchers mound. Everyone was so surprised that no one moved. I was able to pick up the ball and throw it to the catcher for the force at home. Since the batter was still standing there wondering what had happened, the catcher was easily able to throw him out at first base for the third out We eventually won the game.

The second game that I remember was when we left Salinas, California, on completion of my residency. We had driven to Montana to my wife's town, Westby, which was just next to Plentywood. There was the annual Plentywood fastpitch softball tournament starting, and there were teams from Canada and other areas competing. The "Blue Moon" team from Plentywood was short a pitcher. When we went over to watch the games, they heard from Marlene's father that I was a pitcher. They needed a second pitcher for their team, and before you could count to ten, I had been recruited to pitch their second game against one of the really good teams from Regina, Canada. I was not in particularly good shape and had only been playing backyard "catch" for the preceding year. Nevertheless, I started the game and it was a scoreless duel until the fifth inning, when we both scored one run. It went that way until the eleventh inning when we finally scored a run and won the game 2-1. By that time I was going on "fumes" and I doubt that I could have lasted to face another batter. I was so sore the next day that I couldn't lift my arm. The Blue Moon played the rest of the tournament without me. After their other pitcher got a much needed day of rest, they won the tournament.

The last game that I consider memorable was really my "last game." I had stopped pitching and playing in the 1970s. The burden of my medical practice and the constant call and interrupted night's sleep would not let me stay in good enough shape to pitch. In 1996, I was asked if I could still pitch and help out one of the teams in the Billings North Park fastpitch league. That seemed like quite a challenge since I was now 65 and had not pitched in 20 years. I started working out and practicing, and I was able to compete fairly well. However, the 15 strikeouts a game were a thing of the past. My speed had gone down from 70 mph to 55 mph, and my rise just wouldn't break the way it used to do. It was no fun giving up home runs to those strong young players. I did play two seasons. The last game that I pitched was against a team that had beaten us every time, but we were ahead by one run, 3-2. There was a man on third base with their best batter coming up. He had hit the ball out of the park on me before and was anxious to do it again. There was no way I could overpower him, so I had to pitch smart and not just fast. I called the catcher to the mound for a conference. "What do you think we should start with", I asked? "He's set to hit it out of the park, so let him. Give him an inside curve and he'll get around on it and hit it foul", my catcher said. I prayed that I could keep it inside, and sure enough, I broke it inside close to his hands, and he fouled it off, out of the park. "Strike one." Another conference and we decided to give him a change-up. "Be sure to keep it outside and low," he said. I made the pitch look like I gave it everything I had , and he took a mighty swing, but early. "Strike two." Now, things were getting interesting. What to throw next? He would not expect another change-up so that was what I threw. He lunged for the ball that looked like it was coming in fat and just right for a huge hit. The ball fell away as he took his third swing and he got nothing but air. "Strike three." We were out of the inning and still ahead. I left the game and our other pitcher held them for the last 3 innings.

At that point I decided that it was time to stop competing with the 25 year olds, and I turned to coaching girls fastpitch. I actually learned more about proper technique and the mechanics of the pitching delivery than I had known when I was competing. I also worked with the younger 12-14 year old girls who were just learning their fundamentals. This kept me in pretty good shape and surprisingly, the only part of my body that doesn't hurt is my left arm. At age 75, I think longingly, "Could I do it again?" Age and guile still trumps youth and speed, but there is a time when reality sets in. Then it's time to hang up the glove and live with the memories.

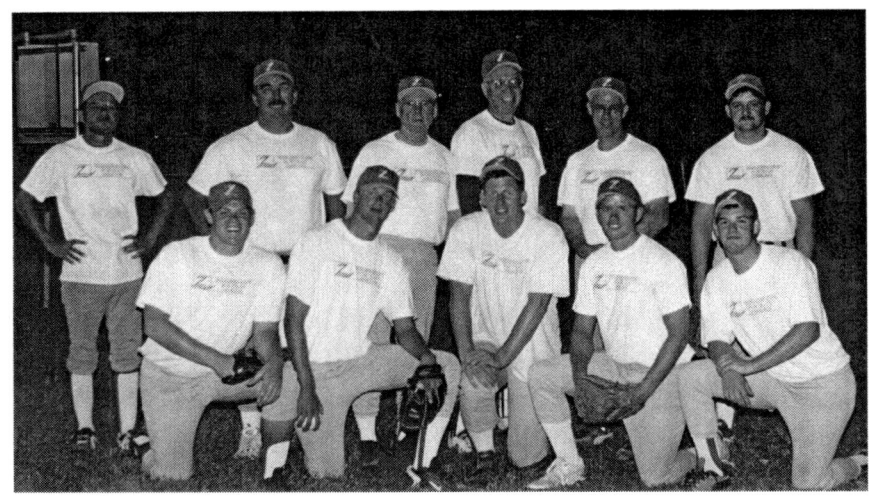

My last team at age 66.

CHAPTER 4
MEDICAL SCHOOL

Needless to say, those of us who applied to Baylor Medical College after just three years of college instead of a four year degree were a little apprehensive of acceptance. But, with good grades, letters of recommendation, and a prestigious college (Rice University) to fortify us, we were hopeful.

We had to have an interview with the Assistant Dean of Baylor, Dr. James Schofield, who was somewhat intimidating. That interview was a little stressful for those of us who had never applied for a spot where there were many more applicants than slots for the freshman class. Dr. Schofield had a "thing" that he included with all of his interviews that I have never really figured out. There were three pictures of clowns on his wall that he would take down and ask us to interpret. One was a happy clown, another a sad clown, and another was a clown with a frown. I don't really remember what I said about them. Today I would probably have said that the first clown was happy that he passed the interview and got into Baylor, and the second was sad because he was rejected. The frowning third clown was wondering if Dr. Schoefield could smell what he was sitting in, due to the stress of the interview.

In any event, all of the Rice applicants were accepted. The first day of orientation, while we sat in the auditorium, was a little unsettling. We were told to look around, and then were told that by mid-year, about twenty percent of us would no longer be there. Fortunately, all of the Rice students made it through, and most were in the top one third in class ranking, since we had been conditioned to study incredibly hard in order to survive our time at Rice. By the end of the first year, however, our standings were scattered randomly, as the rest of the class met the challenge of this degree of commitment to studying.

We were divided into groups of four for the various labs, and then were sent to the anatomy lab to lay claim to one of the tables that held the formaldehyde saturated cadavers. The word was to get a thin male, since that made the dissections easier. I was one of the first to enter the anatomy room and quickly claimed one. I announced to my three other cohorts that I had a thin black male for us. As my friends approached the table, they informed me that although I had picked a thin one, I really needed the anatomy class, since I had picked a flat chested female and didn't seem to know the difference in the sexes.

One of our classmates, Whitney, was the class practical joker. I had been with him in high school and he gave the teachers fits even then. I was a little surprised to see him again in medical school, but he turned out to be a fine student. He eventually became head of the ophthalmology department at Baylor. However, he never lost his flair for practical jokes, and I remember what happened in the anatomy classroom only too well.

Well, the story in anatomy lab goes like this....The girls from the Baptist Student Union at Rice were coming to the medical school, and were going to visit the anatomy lab as part of their tour. Rice campus is only a few blocks from the medical school. Whitney and his anatomy table group planned a little surprise for the naive college girls. His cadaver was a large male who was rather well endowed. Whitney's group took a straight wire probe and catheterized the man's penis to make it stand upright, and then tied a large red ribbon around it. They then waited innocently for the girls to enter the anatomy room. Since their table was nearest the entrance, there was no question as to what would be the first sight encountered. I watched the first three that entered, a cute, bouncy blond, a taller brunette, and a slightly heavy-set girl with glasses. The brunette spied the presentation first, and exclaimed to the blond, "My God, would you look at that? No, stop, don't look at that!" They seemed to be blushing, but maybe it was a reflection from the reddish brown floor. After a few giggles, they made a left turn to avoid that table and proceeded down another aisle on their tour. Needless to say, there were some repercussions and explaining to do in the Dean's office. I would have loved to be a fly in the corner when Whitney gave his version of the incident to the Dean.

We had a visiting professor that year, who would give a short lecture pertaining to the area of study for the day. At the time, I was unable to appreciate the pearls of wisdom that he gave out until years later. When situations would arise that would call back his words, I wish that I had listened more attentively. The time we spent on the inguinal triangle dissection in the groin did not seem to be so important to me then. When I began to repair hernias in my practice, however, those muscles, ligaments, and attachments suddenly took on a new perspective in order for me to plan the type of approach that would be required for each individual case.

Not until I was in practice did I have reason to recall his lecture on the "triangle of death" in the neck. I had a patient with a large boil on his neck which made it a lot more serious than one in another part of the body. Infections involving the veins in that area could extend easily upward into the brain, since there were no valves in the veins of that area to prevent backwash of infected blood and material into the brain. I watched him carefully until it had cleared up completely. Likewise, the complex anatomy of the hand did not really hit me until I had to repair severe hand lacerations with severed tendons. That fact sent me back to the anatomy books for an in-depth-review.

We spent the first six weeks of anatomy class on the lower extremity. We all probably knew the origins and insertions of the thigh muscles better than any other muscles of the body when we finished the course. Years later, that knowledge was still crystal clear in my mind when I had to repair the anterior thigh of a young boy who had somehow dropped a spinning circular saw on his upper leg, and severed most of the anterior compartment of muscles down to the bone. There are a number of muscles in the anterior thigh and after the saw went through them, they did not look like the pictures in the textbook. Nevertheless, I was able to trace out the anatomy, and put the proper ends back together. The surgery went well and he recovered uneventfully. Today, a procedure such as that would not have been repaired by a general practitioner, but would have been referred to a general, or plastic surgeon.

Neuroanatomy was one of the most fascinating courses that we studied, and we had a wonderful professor, Dr. John Perry. By the time we had finished that course of lectures and dissections, we knew every connection, tract, and pathway of the brain. We could pinpoint where each lesion would be, according to the physical findings of the patient. We used to make up scenarios with a number of physical findings to test each other on the location of the brain injury. That knowledge however, didn't stay with me in such detail for very many years since I didn't go into neurosurgery as a specialty. Now, with the ability to use "clot buster" drugs for strokes as well as heart attacks, it again calls up the anatomy of the brain and where the occlusion has occurred.

My work as a laboratory technician became important when we started bacteriology and biochemistry. Tests in those days were not automated as they are today, and they required chemical reactions to produce various colors which could then be read in a colorimeter. They were read after the colorimeter was calibrated using known amounts of glucose, cholesterol, or other blood constituents that were being analyzed. I had been doing that as part of my job in Schulze's lab for several years, as well as the hematology and bacteriology testing and analysis, so that was "old hat" for me.

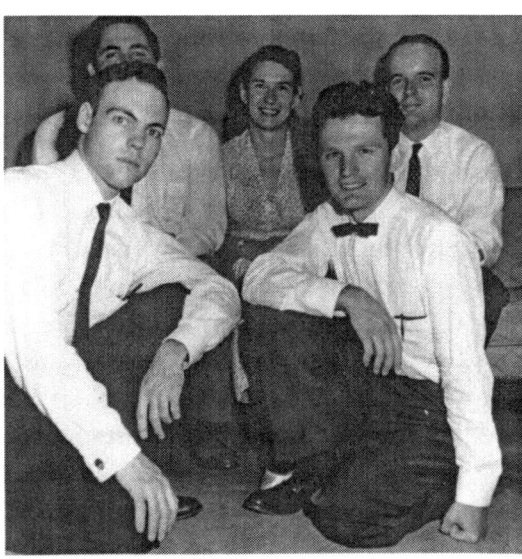

Our lab group, (left to right) Myself, Demitri George, Julie Martin, Sam Luce, Jim McMurtry

In physiology lab we had to do various studies using dogs after they were anesthetized, and subjected to whatever the investigation called for. They were then euthanized at the conclusion of the experiment. Sometimes we had projects that required several days. The dog might be allowed to wake up and then used again until the study was concluded. Our group had selected a problem to investigate that required monitoring the blood sugar after injecting various substances into the dog. Our study required five days to complete so we used the same dog for that investigation. I selected a friendly, black, short haired, duke's mixture for our subject. She almost seemed to look forward to coming with me each day as I brought her down from the roof where all the dogs were kept in penned enclosures. When we finished our tests at the end of the week, I could not bear to send her back to the roof and certain death when she was selected for someone else's study. I told my cohorts, "She's not going back to the roof if I can help it." I looked at her and said, "If I take you back to the roof, your life isn't worth a plugged nickel. Do you want to come home with me?" She looked at me with those soft brown eyes straight into my soul, raised her paw, and said "Woof." At the end of the day, with some stealth, I managed to sneak her out of the school and brought her home. I said to my mother who met us at the back door, "Meet Tollie, the newest addition to our family." Mother was surprised, but Tollie wagged her tail, dribbled a little urine on the kitchen floor in her joy to be out of the medical school, and bonded with her immediately.

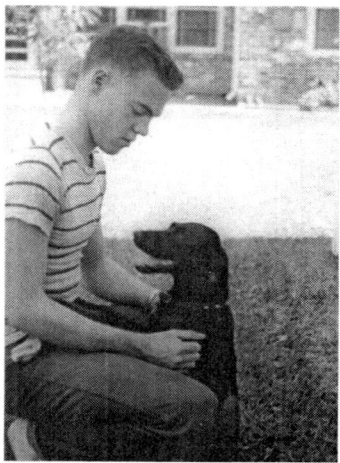

Tollie

She turned out to be one of the nicest pets that one could have. I named her "Tollie" after the glucose tolerance tests that we performed on her. She had one litter of pups, evidently conceived while in captivity at the medical school, and then we had her spayed. Tollie learned quite a repertoire of tricks to impress whoever came to visit, and she enjoyed performing. She became a surrogate child after I graduated and left home. She lived a long, lovable life, finally dying of old age.

Our classes in pathology during our second year reminded me about the great anatomists and pathologists of the past, including Addison (Addison's Disease), Hodgkins (lymph node cancer), Lannec (Cirrhosis), and Virchow (tuberculosis). Peering through the microscope and learning to distinguish the cells of various organs, and then learning to recognize the normal from the abnormal made me realize how far we have come in the last one hundred fifty years. At that time, it was not known what caused people to fall ill and die. It was thought that unseen humors, fluxes, and miasmas would descend on a person and cause an altered state of health, thus causing illness.

There was no thought given to organs becoming diseased and then causing the whole person to become ill as a result, until Rudolph Virchow peered through his microscope and examined various tissues at a cellular level. He could see that diseased cells from organs of sick people looked different than those of healthy persons. Virchow did not receive his medical degree until 1843, when very little was really understood about disease. Within only a few years he, barely a stripling physician, had discovered leukemia, or "white blood disease" as he initially called it. A year later in 1846, he demonstrated the true nature of blood clotting and the difference between thrombosis, where a vessel becomes occluded, and embolus, where a clot breaks away and is carried away to occlude a major vessel in a distant part of the body.

Our pathology instructor, Dr. Stuart Wallace, in his quiet way, instilled in us a desire to understand and recognize the changes that we would see on those slides and not soon forget. I took his teaching to heart, and even when I was in private practice I would enjoy examining slides of the tissues and biopsies that I would send to the pathologist, Dr. Glenn. He knew of my interest and would send me a slide back with the report so that I could examine it myself.

Bacteriology class began in the sophomore year. I had already been doing bacteriology in Schulze's lab, giving me a little more familiarity with picking colonies from culture plates, streaking the plates for isolation of the colonies, and then staining slides from the material for identification. I remember a serious error in my early career at the lab which could have cost me my life. Nowadays we have a hood that shields us from possible spills or contaminations when working with hazardous materials, but there were no such safeguards in place at that time. I was transferring a colony of tuberculosis bacteria from a culture plate to a slide to be stained, and after I made the transfer, I flamed the platinum loop. There was a small pop as the moisture in the colony exploded before it could all be incinerated in the flame. I am sure that I aerosolized about a million bacteria into the air. I didn't think anything about it at the time, but when I had a TB skin test the next year, it had turned from negative to positive. I never became ill, but I evidently developed a primary infection, and then immunity. In those years we were just developing drugs to combat TB, such as streptomycin and paraminobenzoic acid, and these drugs had significant unpleasant side effects. Now, any conversion of a TB test if discovered within one year is routinely treated with INH (isoniazide) for prophylaxis.

Actually, the science of bacteriology is not that old. The thought that germs, those little unseen critters seen under the microscope, could cause disease was first entertained by Dr. Joseph Lister, the father of antiseptic surgery, in 1867. He saw the same germs in autopsy specimens that he saw in infected wounds and made the connection. He knew that carbolic acid was used by sanitation workers to keep the smell in check at the refuse dumps; therefore he decided to spray it in his operating room, and also to place towels soaked in it around the wounds when he was operating. He had read letters from Louis Pasteur, who found in 1865 that organisms could contaminate the fermentation process in wine and beer, and he surmised that these germs could also cause havoc in his surgical patients. He was rewarded with a much lower infection rate and the age of antiseptic surgery was slowly brought onto the scene with much skepticism from his colleagues.

In 1847, Ignac Semmelweis had run up against a similar brick wall as he tried to convince the obstetricians of the day to wash their hands in a chloride of lime solution before attending deliveries. Women would die in large numbers from childbed fever as these physicians unknowingly carried the deadly streptococcus from the autopsy room into the delivery room on their unwashed hands. The nurse-midwives had a much lower infection rate with their deliveries on their wards. They were not permitted to be in the autopsy room and were also much more fastidious with keeping their hands and uniforms clean. The doctors never seemed to make the connection and Semmelweis was completely ridiculed and rejected. He was not very diplomatic in his criticism of his peers, and he cursed them for their stupidity. Eventually he was forced to leave the University of Vienna because of his outlandish theories about childbed fever. It was not until several years later that his students would be able to convince their peers that he was right, and finally they began to wash their hands.

It was not until 1876 that a German bacteriologist, Robert Koch, first proved that specific bacteria could cause a specific illness. He first identified Anthrax, then the streptococcus, staphylococcus, pneumococcus and two other bacilli as causes of specific illnesses. He developed Koch's postulates which consisted of taking material from an infected lab animal, culturing it, instilling the cultured bacteria into another lab animal, producing the same disease, and then recovering the same bacteria. This was dramatic evidence that "germs caused disease." We are not that far removed from the "Cave Man" era.

I can't finish this chapter without mentioning my relationship and friendship with another classmate, Sam Luce. I was still running my band on weekends and I learned that Sam was an accomplished string bass player. I invited him to come play with our three piece, and soon to be, four piece band. The addition of the deep rich sound of a stand up bass was great.

Sam was very innovative, and still had the pioneer and outdoorsman spirit that would continue to dominate his life into the future. In fact, there is a book written about him called "Maverick Doc" that I highly recommend. Sam was a hunter, horseman, and a person who felt that if you could make it yourself, it was better than buying it. He made his own leather pants, boots, and holster for his six-gun, and he reloaded ammo for his pistols and 45/70 buffalo gun.

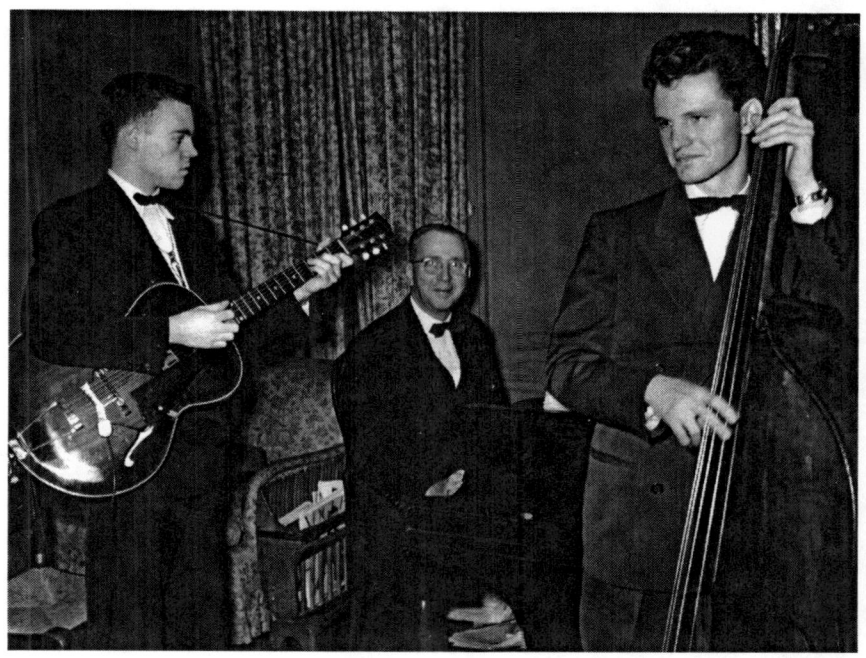

Elmer Schulze, Sam Luce and myself.

I imitated him to a degree. Instead of leather pants, I got my mother to teach me how to cut out a sheepskin coat from a pattern, sew it up and line it with satin. I couldn't let him get too far ahead of me. I got to be a decent holster maker for my numerous pistols that I collected over the years, after Sam showed me how. I got my share of deer, antelope, elk, geese, ducks, and pheasants, but I didn't make it a second profession like he did. After graduation, Sam set up practice in Estes Park, Colorado, where he could take off when the spirit hit him to go hunt mountain lions when the practice got too hectic. He married a classmate, Julia Martin, who shared his love of ranching and the outdoors, and they have remained good friends of mine ever since.

Well, most of us passed through the first two years of lectures and labs, and in our third year, we took physical diagnosis and began to apply the knowledge from the classroom to the human body. The teaching methods have changed now, and physical diagnosis is incorporated earlier, allowing the student to get the "Big Picture" all at once instead of in pieces.

CHAPTER 5
PHYSICAL DIAGNOSIS

Our junior year saw the beginning of clinics. We had finished physical diagnosis at the end of the sophomore year, and now we had to make a visit to a surgical supply house to buy the instruments that we would carry in our medical bags. The day we went to the surgical supply vendors was exciting. Now we could foresee our future with real medical instruments and the opportunity to begin examining live patients with the knowledge that we had been collecting in our brains for the last two years. There was a supply house in the building where Elmer Schulze had the medical lab. With some financial help from him, I purchased my stethoscope, blood pressure cuff, otoscope, ophthalmoscope, tuning fork (to test hearing), head mirror, and reflex hammer. Now, with a white coat and a stethoscope around my neck, I began to feel like a real doctor.

In physical diagnosis we learned to take a history, which included a system review, past and present history, family history, medication history, operations, illnesses, and immunizations. We had to write down every part of our exam, and the adage, "If you didn't write it down, you didn't do it," applied.

At this point, I should digress a bit and talk about three of the newly acquired instruments: the stethoscope, the head mirror, and the blood pressure cuff. These instruments made an enormous impact on the practice of medicine.

Rene Lannec was a practicing physician in France in 1816. The idea of correlating disease with physical symptoms was still in its infancy.

Listening to the various sounds made by the heart, lungs, and abdomen was difficult and sometimes embarrassing, since it required placing one's ear against the chest or abdomen of the patient in order to listen to the noises made by those areas. Lannec had a young woman patient who was quite obese, and she was suffering from some type of heart condition. Placing his ear against her breast was not appropriate due to her modesty. He recalled an instance when he was watching two young boys playing a game in the park by placing an ear to a plank of wood and then scratching out a code at the other end with a pin. The sound was transmitted through the wood to the ear clearly.

I played the same game with two oatmeal cans and a long piece of stretched string to make a primitive telephone when I was young. We would speak on one end, and the sound came out of our improvised telephone at the other end quite clearly.

Lannec tightly rolled up a sheaf of paper and secured it so that there was a small tube and a solid surrounding area. Surprisingly, he was able to hear her heart tones with remarkable clarity. Refinements using wooden cylinders with a hole bored through and a concave end that could be tightly pressed against the skin quickly followed. Several years later, it was converted to enable both ears to be used by fashioning ivory tipped ear pieces and coiled wire covered with cloth and gum elastic with an ebony chest plate. The instrument initially had several names, but using the Greek word stethos, or chest, and skopus, or observer, the instrument was named. Lannec just called it "le cylindre."

Before we had flashlights, it was difficult to examine noses, throats, ears, and internal cavities. Reflecting light from a mirror was not really satisfactory since it did not focus the reflected light very well. But, by using a concave mirror, the light could be both focused and reflected toward its intended object. This, however, was cumbersome and difficult to align with the examiner's eye. Then the simple solution was made to make a smaller concave mirror, cut a hole in the center, and attach it to the examiner's head with a band of leather. One could then look through the hole directly at the target after placing a light source in back of the patient to reflect the light. Suddenly, the specialty of ear, nose, and throat, was born.

Blood pressure was first measured by Stephen Hales, a veterinarian, in 1733. He inserted a brass tube into the neck artery of a horse and then attached it to a long glass tube to measure the height of the column of blood. Until 1616 it was assumed that the heart constantly formed blood that flowed out to the various parts of the body, and was then destroyed. I am sure that the farmers of the day, using common sense, were smarter than the learned medical minds, who were incorrect in so many obvious functions of the body.

Measuring blood pressure in humans was not done until 1847. It was an invasive procedure, performed by inserting a brass cannula into an artery. I certainly would not have liked to have been the patient. In 1855, the noninvasive procedure of using an inflatable cuff to compress the artery was developed. My first sphigmomanometer used a column of mercury to measure the pressure instead of a spring type device that we now use. It was more accurate, and never needed calibrating, but was too cumbersome to carry in a doctor's bag. Blood pressure is still measured in millimeters of mercury today.

Well, we had the tools, knew how to use them, and had physical diagnosis under our belts. It was now time to head out for the clinics and emergency rooms.

CHAPTER 6
THE EMERGENCY ROOM

The emergency department at Jeff Davis County Hospital was always controlled chaos, and sometimes not so controlled. With more patients than could be comfortably cared for, any help was always appreciated. We were given a basic class in suturing techniques, but needed practice to improve our skills. On Saturday night there were always large numbers of fights, stabbings, and razor cuts that required repair, and not enough interns to handle the job. Enter the medical student....

We could always count on plenty of practice in repair of superficial wounds every Saturday. It would inevitably happen that the perpetrator of the wounds one weekend would be the patient to get sutured the next weekend after retaliation had occurred.

I had an interesting lesson about making a thorough evaluation before starting on a patient one Saturday night. My patient had been in a razor fight, and he had sustained multiple cuts by his opponent from his face down to his torso. After the resident physician had evaluated him and determined him stable enough for the medical student, I began my repairs. He had multiple lacerations, so I decided to start on the more distal wounds and work toward the trunk. "Wow! Who did this?" I asked. "You'll find out next week when he's in here," he replied. None of the cuts seemed to be bleeding excessively, so I covered everything with drapes, and then moved my drape with the hole in the center to each wound as I started a new repair. I began to sew up the wounds, one after the other, and most were superficial enough that only skin sutures were required. When, after about an hour and eight repairs completed, I lifted up the drape and I saw a deeper slash on his side that had cut a small artery. It had pumped about two pints of blood onto the gurney cart and down the wall onto the floor, all hidden conveniently by my surgical drapes. I immediately clamped the bleeder, tied it, and completed the repair, but my patient had the appearance of someone who had just been visited by Count Dracula for a long awaited meal. I started with a black man, but he looked whiter after that incident. It's important to examine a patient completely before starting treatment, and that has stayed with me ever since then.

People always seem to be putting things in various orifices of their body after a little too much alcohol. I have seen quite an array of objects in strange places in my time, and I am not talking about in one's ear. Once when I was in the Jefferson Davis County Hospital ER, there were a group of interns and residents clustered around one exam room. The story was that a patient had, in a drunken moment, pushed a light bulb up his rectum. The resident was unable to remove it with several grasping instruments and they were all perplexed as to what to do next. One of our classmates, Liz Muchmore, had very tiny hands, and the suggestion was made that maybe she could get her hand through the sphincter and hook two strings with slipknots onto the narrow end of the light bulb which was facing upstream. Then, with traction on the string, the light bulb could be guided down and out. Well, the patient was given some open drip ether until he was "out" and very relaxed. Liz was then able, after some slow stretching, to get her hand in, slip the strings over the screw end and bring it down where it could be removed without the glass breaking. This proves the adage, "There is a light at the end of the tunnel."

That's not my only story. I was assigned a patient who said that he needed to see a psychiatrist, but first he had a more immediate problem. He had been drinking and playing with his class ring whereby he slipped it over his penis and then passed out until the next morning. Well, by then the swelling was enormous, and it was almost impossible to even find the ring. He was in danger of having circulatory problems in short order. I was finally able to get a glimpse of the gold ring and work a ring cutter underneath it. A few turns of the ring cutter's wheel and I was able to cut through the ring and relieve the constricting effect.

The patient was greatly relieved, but I don't know if he ever saw the psychiatrist.

The last strange object occurred during my first year in Hardin. A cowboy came in complaining of abdominal pain after he and several of his buddies had been drinking the night before. When I palpated his abdomen, I felt a strange tubular mass in his lower left quadrant. Not knowing what this was, I told him I would have to examine his lower colon with my rigid (not like the nice flexible scopes that we have now) sigmoidoscope. When I had gotten the scope in place, I saw something but I wasn't really sure just what I was seeing. It was a hard object. I felt safe grasping it with a long biopsy forceps and then slowly withdrawing everything (scope and grasped foreign body) together so as to not lose my grip. What I found was a twelve inch piece of broomstick. Evidently he had taken a bet that he could insert it all the way and he won. The medical bill, however, was probably more that what he collected on the bet.

Many of the ER patients required emergency surgery because of trauma, gunshot wounds, bleeding ulcers, or something as mundane as acute appendicitis. We were frequently pressed into service as these patients were taken to surgery. Although we would get a formal rotation through surgery later, we learned ahead of time how to scrub, gown, and glove for the sterile operating room. We would only be second assistants for the operations, and as such, we just held retractors and could not really see what was going on deep in the operative field. I remember once, at about 2 A.M. after holding a retractor for about an hour and not getting to see much to keep me interested, I fell asleep for a few minutes standing up. I guess no one noticed, and the surgeon just readjusted my retractor when it got a little loose, and that woke me up.

We got some experience with medical patients in the ER also, but those exams were mostly in conjunction with the intern or resident. We would be shown interesting findings and then be quizzed on the various differential diagnoses. Likewise, with orthopedic patients, we would help with fractures and learn how to apply casting material so it would not be a complete surprise when we took our orthopedic rotation. Going to the ER was not required, but it did provide us with a little more experience earlier in our careers.

CHAPTER 7
CLINICS

Our obstetrical experience was perhaps the best "hands on" rotation that we had. The maternity service at Jefferson Davis County Hospital was extremely busy, so we all got to do a lot of deliveries. Saddle block anesthesia, a type of limited spinal anesthesia, was popular in those days. We got a lot of practice, under the watchful eye of the resident physicians, in carefully placing the needle into the proper interspace in the spine to instill the anesthetic. This helped also when we were on medicine rotation for doing spinal taps, when we suspected meningitis. Once a patient had been given a saddle block, her ability to push was reduced, so forceps delivery was frequently necessary. I was well-trained as a medical student in the application and use of forceps. Many students do not usually get that experience until they become obstetrical residents. I performed eleven deliveries during my rotation, six of which were with the use of forceps.

We scrubbed on C-sections, but our other female surgery experience was reserved for our gynecology rotation. We did get exposure in treating toxemia of pregnancy, which was poorly understood and poorly treated in the 1950s. We were limited in the type of drugs that were available to reduce the blood pressure. The main treatment was bed rest, sedation, salt restriction, and consideration of inducing labor if the baby was sufficiently mature. It had a better chance of survival outside rather than inside the womb.

The cure of toxemia was delivery, and within hours or a few days, the blood pressure would decrease, diuresis would occur, and blood flow to the kidneys would dramatically improve. It is not my idea here to deliver a lecture on preclampsia, but just to mention some of the information that was known at the time. We still use the general measures noted above and still incorporate magnesium sulfate, narcotics, and sedatives in the treatment. Paraldehyde, used extensively in the 1950s for sedation, has disappeared, in addition to veratrum veride, phenobarbital, ammonium chloride, apresoline, and reserpine.

Women in the county hospital culture did not always come in for regular prenatal care where early signs of toxemia could be recognized and treatment could be started early. They frequently presented when the symptoms were more advance and serious. Likewise, many were seen for the first time when they were in active labor for their pregnancies.

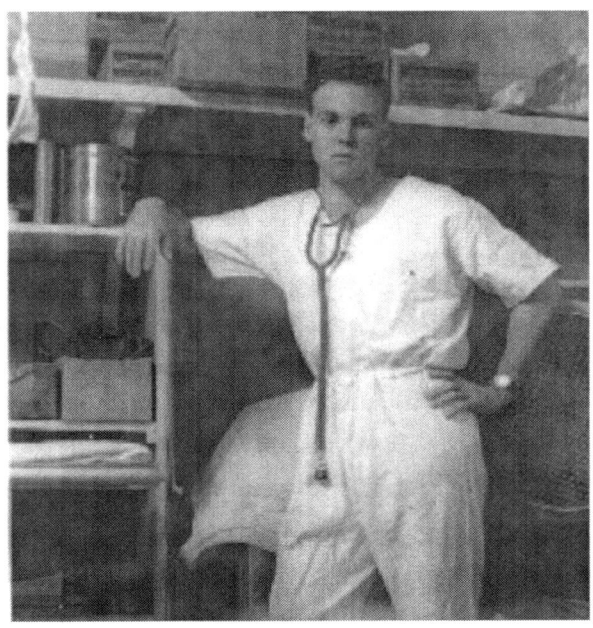

Obstetrical Service at Jefferson Davis Hospital

On pediatric clinic rotation, almost all of us got sick with one of the many viruses that the snotty- nosed kids presented, despite trying to wash our hands as much as possible. After a few weeks, we were mostly immune. Serious problems, such as whooping cough, epiglotitis, measles, chicken pox, mumps, and German measles, were common, since the children of that era did not have the advantage of the preventative immunizations that we have today. Penicillin, sulfa, chloromycetin, and streptomycin were our main drugs to treat most of the infectious diseases of the day.

Polio was a dangerous disease, and I spent some time during that rotation in the polio wards, where the "iron lungs" were breathing for the patients who had the bulbar form of the disease. I am reminded of how lucky I was to get through that era unscathed.

When I was a boy scout at about the age of fourteen, I was at scout camp with my close friend, Herb Schaumburg. He became ill with fever, aching, malaise, and generally being sick. We were sleeping next to each other in the same tent, so I was giving him aspirin and having him drink out of my canteen in the prodromal part of his illness. When he became sicker, he was taken home and hospitalized with paralytic polio. He was severely stricken, and was left with significant weakness and some permanent loss of function. Despite this disability, he later went to medical school. He became one of the world's outstanding neurotoxicologists and is a longstanding department head at Albert Einstein College of Medicine.

During one of my pediatric clinic days, a family of three young children was present, with one being ill with a respiratory illness. One of the youngsters was inquisitive when I was using my stethoscope, and he asked what I was doing. I told him that I was listening to his brother's heart, and would he like to listen to his own heartbeat? I gave him my stethoscope and said, "Do you hear it go lub dub, lub dub?" "No", he said, "It goes ding-a-ling." I took my stethoscope back from him and placed it on his chest. To my surprise, a loud congenital heart murmur was present. His mother was not aware that anyone had ever mentioned anything to her before. He had never really been examined, since he had avoided being sick enough to warrant a visit to the doctor during his five years of life. He was immediately referred upstairs to the pediatric cardiology service. I never heard how things turned out, but in those days, heart surgery was in its infancy. The heart-lung machine was just being developed, and the pioneers of cardiac surgery, Dr. Michael Debakey, and Dr. Denton Cooley, were both at our medical school and at the forefront of this new advancement.

Dermatology clinic was everybody's favorite. We had an excellent professor, Dr. John Knox. I think about half the class wanted to be dermatologists after that rotation. We got to see a large variety of skin afflictions, and after making our evaluation, he, or one of the residents would evaluate our findings and plan of treatment. Because we didn't have cortisone cream or pills in those days, a lot of compounded ointments were used. These included menthol and phenol cream for chronic dermatitis, calomel, and Whitfield's ointment (a mixture of benzoic and salicylic acids) which effectively cured most ringworm and "jock itch." Gentian Violet painted on oral thrush (yeast infection of babies' mouths), and potassium permanganate solution used for athlete's foot were as good as anything we have today but are no longer readily available. This is probably because they are not commercially profitable for the drug companies. Scabies was treated with benzyl benzoate, but it is considered too toxic in today's armamentarium, as are merthiolate and mercurochrome, which both contain mercury. Yellow oxide of mercury was a great ointment for eye infections but that is also gone. We treated warts with a variety of medicines, but would usually burn them off with an electric needle. We didn't have access to liquid nitrogen in those days, which is a much superior treatment.

All of these clinics gradually exposed us to an ever expanding variety of diseases, and we were now ready to enter our senior year.

CHAPTER 8
YELLOWSTONE PARK

There are a few encounters in our lives that seem insignificant at first glance, but are life changing events. The first for me was my chance meeting with Elmer Schulze. If you remember, I was hitchhiking home from high school and got the ride home that started me down the path of my medical career. The second was a chance stroll down the hall of the VA hospital in Houston, on my way to a lecture on tuberculosis. I was walking with a senior medical student who was also attending the lecture, and somehow we began talking about Yellowstone Park. I said that since visiting it a number of years ago, I had always wanted to work there during the summer break from school. He told me that he had worked there at the end of his junior year as an "extern" at the Park Hospital, and had gotten a lot of good experience. Externs are medical students who have not graduated, but perform a preceptorship under the direction and supervision of the physicians at the hospital. It's sort of like being an intern but without the MD after your name. He said he would write the doctors in Livingston, Montana, and recommend that they hire me for the summer. There were four doctors from Livingston, Drs. Lueck, Pearson, Clemons, and Baskett, who took turns coming to the hospital for a week out of each month to provide medical services. There was also a physician, Dr. Frank Brosius, who had been an extern the summer of 1948, and worked as a physician in the park for two summers and one winter before specializing in cardiology. Well, needless to say, I got the job, and at the end of classes in May, I was off to Yellowstone Park in my old 1949 Plymouth for my first adventure away from home.

Park Hospital was an old structure, and was built by the Army in 1911. Mammoth at that time was called Fort Yellowstone, and the Army was in charge until the National Park Service was formed in about 1920. The hospital was actually a residence, but was later converted to a hospital of sorts. It was severely damaged in the earthquake of 1959 and the new hospital was then built at Lake, which was more centrally located for the Park visitors. The old structure had three stories, the first of which was the living quarters for whichever doctor was there during his rotation. There was a kitchen and staff dining room, a business office, a small lab, pharmacy, and several exam rooms to treat patients. The second floor had patient wards, the operating room, nurse's station, medicine closet, and a somewhat primitive central supply. The third floor was for the nurses' residence and externs' quarters.

After getting settled in, I was introduced to the staff and some of the nurses. The hospital was just in the process of opening for the formal tourist season, and all the nurses had not yet arrived. The other extern, Harvey, had not arrived, so I was alone on clinic duty with Dr. Brosius as my preceptor. Things weren't quite as formal and uptight in those days. Since medical malpractice was not much of an issue, I was turned loose to see patients and was to call Dr. Brosius if I had a problem. They did not have much in the way of a clinical lab, so I helped in setting up measures to do blood counts, urinalysis testing, and microscopy. Fortunately, I had brought my microscope with me from Texas, along with the blood testing supplies, pipettes, and counting chamber for the white blood and red blood cell counts.

Most of the medical visits were for things like tonsillitis, ear infections, bronchitis, diarrhea, minor injuries, sprains and a few lacerations. The bears were not restrained from the roads where they would beg for food, and many of the tourists did not realize that these were wild, dangerous animals. The tourists would frequently get out of their cars to feed the bears and have their pictures taken. This resulted in a number of bear bites, some of which were quite severe. I think I repaired about a dozen bear injuries that summer, and some were complex wounds requiring everything I had been taught about how to perform a debridement, and a layered wound closure.

Dr. Brosius watched me quite closely for the first few repairs, but then just inspected the final result after that. I did lab work for the doctors, and they thought it was great to be able to get a blood count, urinalysis, or stained bacterial slides of throats or other areas. We got some blood typing serum at my request and I cross matched blood on two occasions from the walking blood bank, when we got a patient who had a bleeding ulcer, and another who was bleeding from an injury.

There was one occasion when there was a surgical emergency and Dr. Lueck, the surgeon, was there. They did not have an anesthetist on the staff, so I stepped up and told them that I had just finished my anesthesia rotation a few weeks earlier, and that I could drip ether. Because of medical malpractice, no one in this day would consider letting a medical student who had just shown up for work, and had yet to prove himself, handle the anesthesia, but in collaboration with one of the other doctors, I did the anesthesia on that case, and things went OK.

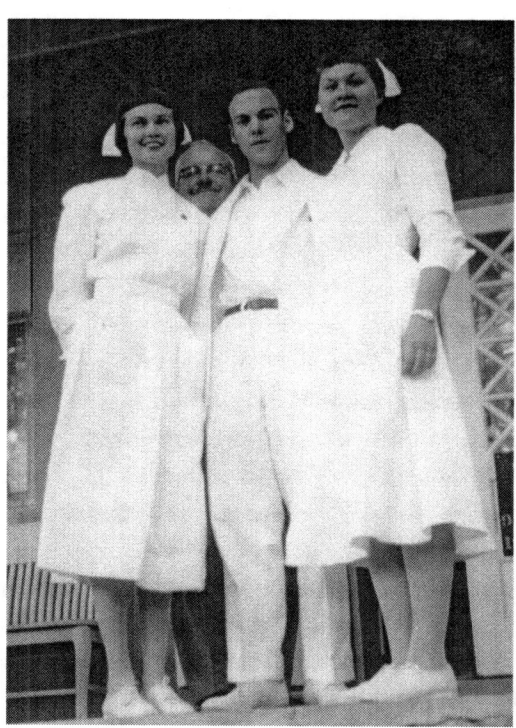

Rose, Dr. Lueck, myself and Shirley.

Ether is a very safe anesthetic, although it is explosive and causes postoperative nausea. There are stages, or depths of anesthesia using ether that one can measure, such as pupil dilation, depth of breathing, blood pressure, pulse, and muscular relaxation. The depth of anesthesia can be regulated just by removing the ether mask for a few minutes, or, if the ether is being volatilized in an oxygen cannister and bag, the amount can be decreased or shut off. Because of the two side effects listed above, we don't use it any more, but in 1956 it still enjoyed a spot in our armamentarium along with pentathol, Demoral, and muscle relaxants.

At this point, perhaps a history lesson on the advent of anesthesia is in order. Prior to the mid 1840s, surgery was performed mostly with nothing more than whisky, laudanum, and several strong men to hold the patient down. Ether had been discovered in the 1600s but it was more of a medical curiosity, and no medical uses were envisioned. Because it was known that if you sniffed it, you would get giddy and act silly, there were parties called ether frolics, where the guests would breathe a few whiffs and behave in an uninhibited fashion to everyone's amusement.

The story goes that at one of these parties was a dentist, Dr. William Morton. He noted that one of the guests had vigorously breathed the sulfuric ether, staggered, and had fallen, cutting his leg in the process. The other guests questioned him about the pain associated with the injury after he had recovered from the ether effects. He denied any pain and had very little recollection of the incident. Dr. Morton, upon observing the incident, thought that he might induce the same state of inebriation for his patients and perform a dental extraction painlessly in the process. It worked well, and encouraged by this, he persuaded a surgeon, Dr. John Warren to perform the first public demonstration of surgery under this new innovation on October 16, 1846, at the Massachusetts General Hospital. Dr. Morton was late for the surgery, and Dr. Warren was about to begin the operation without the benefit of anesthesia, when Morton finally arrived with his ether apparatus. There were comments from the gallery about crazy new fangled ideas as he anesthetized the patient, but soon the patient was asleep. "He is ready for you to proceed, Dr. Warren," Morton announced. There were now murmurs from the gallery as the patient remained asleep. A congenital tumor on the side of the neck of Gilbott Abbott was removed successfully, without pain, in a thirty minute operation. Dr Warren looked up at the gallery and said, "Doctors, This ether thing that we have seen is no humbug." This news spread like wildfire throughout the world in a matter of weeks. The era of painless surgery had arrived. Other volatile liquids were also tried, but chloroform proved to be the best of these other compounds. It was considerably more potent than ether and was non explosive. It was used a lot in obstetrics in those early days since no one at that time knew that it was quite toxic to the liver.

One should not be too smug about thinking that he knows all the answers, because sometimes someone will prove that person wrong, as this next story demonstrates. I was on duty when a Park Ranger came to the hospital and said there was an elderly man at the hotel who was behaving in a bizarre manner. He needed someone from the hospital to evaluate the man. I had just been on the psychiatric service toward the end of the medical school year and had to deal with numerous schizophrenics, both of the catatonic and paranoid types. I was still thinking in that vein when I began to try to examine this man, and get him to calm down and sit down. He made no sense and I began to think he was having some sort of "nervous breakdown" until a bellhop walked by and said, "That man is in diabetic shock and needs some orange juice," which he promptly went to get. He got him to drink the orange juice with sugar, and in a few minutes, as the man's blood sugar began to rise to normal levels, the psychiatric emergency disappeared. The bell hop was a diabetic and was able to recognize the problem immediately. I had never seen anyone with a low blood sugar reaction in my young career. I congratulated him on his astute diagnosis, and tucked the information away in my brain for future use. Fortunately, I kept my mouth closed long enough so that I didn't put my foot in it. I certainly learned a lesson in humility from that experience.

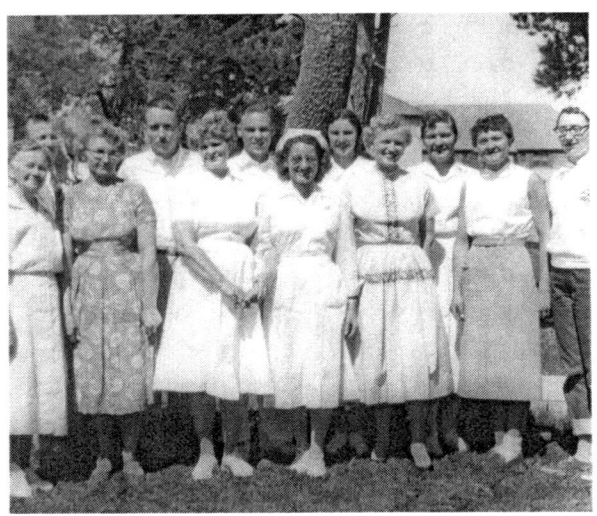

Park Hospital medical staff, 1956.

Those three months at the Park Hospital provided me with a wealth of learning and practical experience from the doctors there. I learned how to read an EKG from Dr. Clemons and Dr. Brosius, and how to interpret all those little squiggles on the paper. That was very helpful later, when we had a formal course in EKG interpretation, since I already had the background in place.

On another unrelated note, I still remember one patient who presented to me with a case of bronchitis. When I had his shirt off and was listening to his lungs, I noted an irregular black mole on his right shoulder which I recognized almost certainly to be a melanoma. We had been lectured about this type of skin cancer in the dermatology clinic. I told him that this mole certainly looked serious to me, and that he should have this taken care of immediately. He made light of it despite my warning, and said that he had the mole for a long time and was not concerned. Malignant melanomas metastasize early. I still wonder if he changed his mind later and had further evaluation, for if he didn't, I am certain he would have paid with his life.

Fishing was very popular in the park, especially fly fishing. At Fishing Bridge there could be dozens of fishermen in close proximity casting

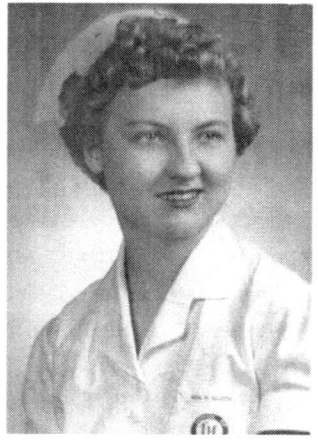

into the water for trout. Naturally, fishhooks were a problem, and I spent a lot of time learning how best to remove a fishhook that had hooked a tourist and not a fish. I remember one patient who was standing close to the bridge talking to a friend, and as he opened his mouth to speak, he got hooked in the tongue by someone's fly hook. I had to anesthetize his tongue, push it through, cut the hook and then grab the barb and pull it the rest of the way out. I have heard of opening your mouth and putting your foot in it, or so the saying goes, but that was ridiculous.

Marlene Nelson

Working at the Park Hospital was where I met my soon to be wife, Marlene Nelson. She had graduated from nursing, and after working at Sidney Montana and Fort Harrison, had decided to take the summer off from nursing and work in the park at Old Faithful as a sales clerk. Several of the nurses who had applied for the nursing positions had failed to show up, so they were short two nurses. The director of nurses at the hospital heard that there were two nurses working as clerks at

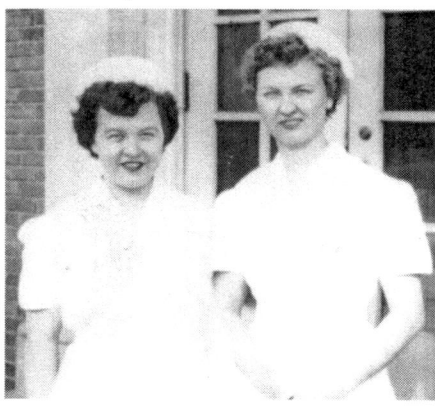

Old Faithful, and she persuaded them to come up to Mammoth and fill the vacancies. So, Marlene and her cousin Jane Nielson, also from Westby, joined the hospital staff.

It was apparent from the start that Marlene was not only the prettiest of all the nurses, but was also a dynamo when it came to working. She got her jobs done and anyone else's who was

Jane Nielsen and Marlene

behind in their work. I knew I would have to convince her to come to Houston after the summer so that I would not lose contact with her. It worked, and she came to Houston and worked at Memorial Hospital during my senior year. We got married after I graduated in June, in her home town of Westby, and she has been my partner ever since.

There was an incident that occurred at Old Faithful that was humorous and yet sad at the same time. Evidently a tourist had something happen to him at the Old Faithful Inn and was pronounced dead. Grant, our handyman and ambulance driver was dispatched to take the body to Livingston in the station wagon ambulance. Grant was somewhat superstitious and really did not like to be around dead people, but his job was to drive the ambulance. It was a stormy, rainy night, and in the middle of the trip, the supposedly dead person sat up in the back of the ambulance and made some sounds. Grant was so frightened by the event that he stopped the ambulance, jumped out in the rain and ran down the highway before he summoned up enough courage to go back to check. I never heard exactly what the patient's outcome was on arrival in Livingston, but Grant was shaken up for days.

Finally, the time had come to return to Houston and start the senior year. I said my goodbyes to all the wonderful people at the hospital, and made Marlene promise to write and consider coming to Houston, and then got in my old Plymouth and headed south.

CHAPTER 9
THE SENIOR YEAR

In our senior year we began inpatient care on each of the major branches of medicine, namely surgery, pediatrics, internal medicine, gynecology, orthopedics, and Dr. Debakey's cardiac surgery. We worked at Jeff Davis Hospital for the majority of these rotations, but switched to the private hospitals, such as Methodist, Texas Children's, and Hermann hospitals, where we worked up some private patients as well. At Jeff Davis, we also spent some time on the psychiatric, the polio, and the tuberculosis wards.

On each service it was the medical student's job to come early and draw all the blood on the ward before rounds started, which was usually at eight o'clock. This was somewhat of a pain if the student was not very good at drawing blood, but one has to learn sometime. I had been drawing blood in the lab for several years and had gotten pretty good at it. If there was a hard draw, I usually helped out that student in our group.

All this blood drawing prompted two medical students at Chapel Hills Medical School to write a song called "Exsanguination Blues," and the lyrics went something like this:

> Now up 'til this year I managed to pass, and never went to an eight o'clock class; why go to class if you like your sleepin' better.
> But this September the worm she turned, 'cause a new kinda routine had to be learned, and I became a bona fide blood-letter.

Now I'm at the hospital way before eight, I have to get there
and exsanguinate; I tell you folks this life can get you down.
There's a BUN and a CBC, a blood sugar and a BSP, a
cholesterol, Na, K, and CO2.
But the thing guaranteed to make you sore, is you gotta look
on every floor,
to find a syringe and needle near the right size.
So you spend thirty minutes gouging for a vein, the patient's
lying there wracked with pain; for miles around you can hear
his pitiful cry.
But you finally get the blood and you get it under oil, and head
for the lab like it was gonna spoil,
and by the clock you see you're done outa' time.
You go runnin' down the hall and around the curve,
the girl sees you comin' and says you got your nerve,
Don't you see, boy, it's way past the deadline.
But a little smile comes over your face,
'cause you got a hole card and it's an ace;
you tell her it's something special for the chief of staff.

That was the first verse, but you get the idea.

Our medicine rotation really brought us into contact for the first
time with seriously ill patients and many conditions that rarely make
themselves known in a routine practice. Our drugs were much
more limited in the late 1950s. Cardiac drugs and antihypertensive
medications could practically be counted on one hand. We had
powdered whole leaf digitalis to help strengthen and slow the heart,
ammonium chloride and aminophylline to help with diuresis, and a
very potent but somewhat toxic injectable diuretic called mercuhydrin,
which contained, you guessed it, mercury. This sort of poisoned the
kidneys and let the fluid run through. We didn't have good enough
tests to see how much damage we were doing to the kidneys, but the
seriousness of the heart failure took center stage at that point, and
the murcuhydrin really worked. We had a few ganglionic blocking
antihypertensives and also Rauwolfia Serpentina or Indian Snake Root,
that worked fairly well, but they made the patients sleepy and depressed.
We did have nitroglycerine for chest pain, but nothing much else for

angina or acute heart attacks except morphine and oxygen. We didn't know about the benefits of aspirin then, nor the use of intravenous lidocaine for the arrhythmias accompanying a heart attack.

Since we didn't have monitors, we didn't really get to see the arrhythmias when they were happening.

Congestive heart failure, especially the acute phase, was treated with rotating tourniquets and phlebotomy (removal) of one unit of blood to prevent the return and overloading of the blood into the right ventricle. Oxygen, morphine, digoxin, and elevation of the patient's head rounded out the treatment.

It is surprising how even in a seriously sick patient, sex is important. I remember an anecdote that happened to one of my patients who had pretty severe chronic congestive heart failure. There were usually four beds to a room with only a curtain separating them. I was examining him with his petite little wife sitting by his side, since he was somewhat critical. I left for lunch and as I was walking through the emergency room I saw her getting her head stitched up. The story was that they had decided to get amorous and she got bounced off the bed and onto the floor, head first. I said to him, "What was going on? "Well Doc," he said, still slightly out of breath, "you gotta do what you gotta do!" Maybe he wasn't as sick as I thought.

With so much material to memorize about all of the diseases that we encountered, we all carried a little book in our white coats, where we kept our notes. There was also the Merck Manual, a very condensed version of most of the medical conditions. It was written in small print and thin paper so it could fit in your coat pocket. The professors didn't like to see us with it since the information was not complete enough and they wanted us to use our large textbooks of medicine.

One day we had been studying strokes and the blood vessels at the base of the brain called the Circle of Willis. Sometimes, there could be a pulsating of blood simulating a thumping or "wumping" sound that the patient perceived. So, one of our group made up a new name, the "Wump" syndrome. A late comer to the group discussion arrived, and wanted to know what that was all about. Woody Woodward, the instigator, with tongue in cheek, told Charlie, the latecomer, that this "Wump Syndrome" was caused by a fecalith, (a calcified piece of poop) rotating around in the Circle of Willis (in the brain) and every time it made the rotation, it went wump! The next day we were making rounds with one of the professors, and were gathered around a patient who had a noise in his head. Well, Charlie was trying to review some information about strokes in his Merck Manual under the patient's bed. The professor, seeing that Charlie was reading out of the "banned book," asked him about the patient's complaint. Charlie, with his newly acquired knowledge from the day before proudly stated that the patient probably had the "Wump syndrome." "What in the world is that?" asked the professor. Charlie told him that it was due to a fecalith swirling around in the Circle of Willis. "Son," said the professor, "Someone is severely pulling your leg!" We could all barely contain ourselves since we had set Charlie up for that encounter.

Blood was always in short supply because of all of the trauma, gunshots, and accidents that were seen by the emergency room. In order to keep up the blood supply available for elective surgery, each service had to get the interns and medical students to recruit relatives of the patients to donate blood so that their relatives could have surgery. There was a rule on the obstetrical service that every pregnant woman had to get one pint of blood donated by someone before she delivered. We would have to paint a picture that all of the patients would actually need the blood that was donated on their behalf. Occasionally, a relative would ask when their family member was going to get the blood that we assured them would be needed. One resourceful intern figured out how to resolve that question. He got some red dye and added it to the IV bottle of glucose to prove that the patient was getting the required blood. I am sure that would probably generate a lawsuit in today's medical climate.

Psychiatric drugs to treat schizophrenia were just becoming available in the mid-1950s. Chlorpromazine was the first, and it made a tremendous step forward in the treatment of hallucinations, voices in the head, and the severe withdrawal of some of the catatonic patients. These patients were locked away in pretty dismal surroundings. The rooms were reminiscent of the "mad houses" of the fifteenth century. They were dismal, poorly lighted, and had bars on the doors and windows. Interviewing these patients and doing their physicals was a little scary for us as medical students, since some patients could become violent due to their illness. The chlorpromazine was able to control their hallucinations for the most part, but large doses were required which made the patients lethargic, and many developed a tremor as a side effect of the medicine, which required other medications to treat these side effects.

Working in the polio wards was somewhat depressing. There were a number of patients in the "iron lungs" which created an alternating positive and negative pressure to allow the patient's lungs to be ventilated. All of their care had to be given with them still in the iron lung. Portals were present for the nurses to insert their hands for changing their clothing, personal care, and bathing. This phase of polio treatment was really time consuming, as was physical therapy to rehabilitate the withered limbs and weakened muscles of respiration. The advent of polio vaccine in the 1950s was one of the most important advances in medicine, but more about that later.

Baylor in the late 1950s was the center of cardiovascular surgery, with the two superstars, Dr. Michael DeBakey and Dr. Denton Cooley. They were the innovators of new and radical procedures to bring healing to the hearts of these doomed patients who arrived from not only the United States, but from all over the world. We all were assigned to Dr. DeBakey's service in groups of six or eight and we had to work up some of these patients in addition to others on the surgical service.

Dr. DeBakey would make rounds on his patients each afternoon with an entourage of resident and interns. Trailing behind in the rear were the medical students. We had a great deal of work ahead of us each afternoon and would have to sit and wait for his rounds which were supposed to begin promptly at 4 P.M. He would frequently be late by as much as forty-five minutes, and that was time we could hardly spare. We did not gain much from the rounds anyway, so our group did the unthinkable. We decided to wait thirty minutes according to protocol, and if he was not there, we would leave, go about our duties, and not trail behind like baby ducks following their mother. Well, it happened, and when he arrived, there were no medical students.

This created a situation that had never happened before, and he was somewhat taken aback. I think this even got reported to the Dean. We stood our ground according to the thirty minute rule, and, at least for the rest of our rotation, he was on time with his rounds.

We did get to scrub on some of the cases as third or fourth assistant and on one occasion Woody Woodward, one of the students, was removing the towel clips that held the skin towels in place at the edge of the incision during the wound closure. The towel clips were opened, disengaged from the patient's skin and then closed and handed to the surgical nurse. Just as Woody was closing the towel clip, Dr. DeBakey reached over to remove the towel from the wound area, and, you guessed it, Woody closed the towel clip through Dr. DeBakey's finger. There were probably a few loud exclamations and apologies after that, so, at the senior banquet, Dr. DeBakey was presented with a Purple Heart towel clip medal, and Woody was presented with an award for extreme valor and bravery.

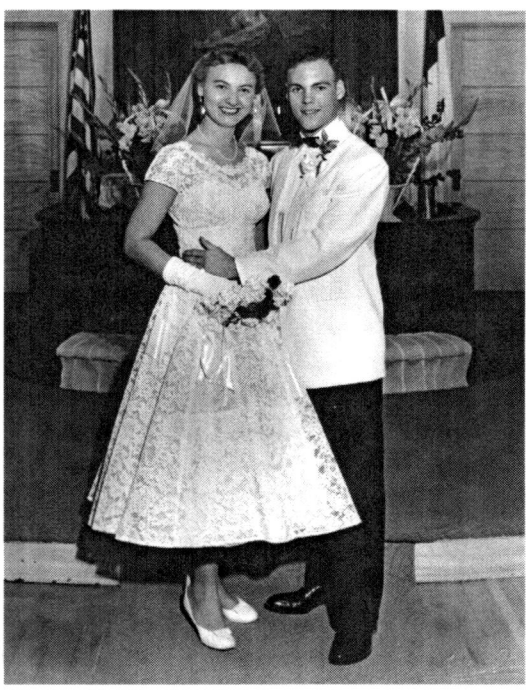

Our wedding in Westby Montana, June 12, 1957.

During my senior year, I had convinced Marlene to move down to Houston, and she got a job at Memorial Hospital. I was sure that she was the one with whom I wanted to share my life. As the months progressed, we became engaged, and planned a wedding when I graduated in June. Ever since we met in Yellowstone Park, a poem had been circulating around in the neurons of my brain, and on our second anniversary I finally got around to writing it down. Poetry is not really my forte, but here is the poem that I wrote to her for that anniversary.

TO MY WIFE ON OUR SECOND ANNIVERSARY

Let me tell you of the story
That to me is very dear.
Of my one true love, my only love,
Now and throughout the years.

We met one day and quite by chance,
In the land called Yellowstone.
And I knew my search was ended,
And I never more would roam.

The days flew by and with each one,
Our summer grew too short.
For with the end I did not know
If we would have to part.

I told her that I loved her,
She said she loved me too.
And when I left that she would follow
In a month or two.

My heart was light and yet so sad,
To leave my love at all.
But one thought cheered me constantly,
She'd come in early fall.

The fall was here, the winter nigh,
The winds blew strong and cold.

And yet no love to comfort me,
No one for me to hold.

The winter passed, the spring appeared,
I waited patiently.
And I began to wonder if
our love was still to be.

And then the day at last did come,
And now my love was here.
My head was light, my mind awhirl,
My heart was filled with cheer.

At last she said she'd marry me,
We planned for early June.
The days were short and life was sweet,
And beautiful the moon.

The day had come, we pledged our love,
To God from whence we came.
And vowed that we would honor, love,
And give thanks to his name.

And now the years have grown to two,
Our love is strong and fast.
And if we live a hundred more,
I know our love will last.

So thus I say a prayer when,
I think of Yellowstone.
For there my quest was ended,
And I never more need roam.

Marlene was not afraid to tackle any job or situation and a good example of that was when a purse snatcher got her purse. She owned a 1955 maroon and white Chevy, her pride and joy, and had been out with several of her nurse friends to a movie. She had dropped them off at the nurses' residence and then parked her car in the lot. As she was walking toward the hospital she noticed a burley, pocked marked, black man walking toward her on the sidewalk. He was looking her up and down and a warning feeling went off inside her. She thought of crossing the street to avoid him but decided against it. She had her clutch bag under her arm containing her car keys, her driver's license and her wallet. As he walked past her, he grabbed the purse from under her arm and started to run. He was short and stocky and Marlene could run faster than he could. She soon caught him and grabbed the edge of his jacket. Her rather tight skirt split all the way up the side as she was chasing him. She held on to his coat for a little while longer during the chase, and between gasps of air said something regarding his mother's marital status. Just then she stumbled in her high heels that she was wearing and lost her grip on his coat. He added speed to his gait with this bit of good luck and got away. In retrospect, I suppose that was a good thing. She said she had no fear of what might have transpired if she had caught him. I guess he was lucky that she was wearing high heels, since she was ready to fight for her car keys, no holds bared. Marlene had to get the police to the scene and have her car towed away until the locks on her car could be changed. They had her look at a few pictures in the "mug book" down at the station but his picture was not there. What an introduction to Houston! But that was not all of her surprises that were yet to come.

Marlene had come from a northern state, Montana. She had not been exposed to racism and prejudice as was currently practiced in the South in the 1950s, so I have to tell you of one of her other experiences. She had gone shopping at Foley's and had become thirsty, so she headed for the water fountain. Above one of the drinking fountains was the word "Colored." "That's funny," she thought. "Why would they color the water?" Then she saw the other fountain that said "White," and realized the implication. When she was through shopping, and loaded down with packages, she got on the bus. She noted that the only empty seats were in the back, so she proceeded there and sat down. Immediately the bus driver stopped the bus, and walked to the back of the bus where she was seated. He told her that she would have to move to the front and stand, since she could not sit with the coloreds in the back. She was forced to straddle a package between her legs, with the others draped over both arms while she hung on to the overhead strap. This was her first exposure to the bigotry that still existed at the time.

The time had now come to start applying for internship positions. I was looking for one that offered plenty of experience. I applied to Cook County in Chicago, Wayne County in Michigan, and San Francisco County in California. I was accepted for a position at San Francisco County Hospital with a salary of $150.00 a month. Fortunately, Marlene could get a job at a livable wage at Southern Pacific Hospital for $450.00 a month, and with that, and careful management of our expenses, we felt we could make ends meet.

Our wedding was planned for June 12, in Westby, Montana. Marlene left to go home and make preparations in the latter part of May. My parents and I traveled to Montana shortly after the medical school graduation ceremony, and soon we were meeting all of her relatives and friends in the few days before the wedding. It was held in the small Lutheran church there. Most of the town turned out, and a great time was had by all. After our wedding, it was back to Houston, to start studying for the State Boards held in Austin, in order to get my Texas license. After the State Board exam, we would head out to San Francisco for the next great adventure of our young lives. No time for a honeymoon, except the three days it took to drive back to Houston from Westby.

CHAPTER 10
SAN FRANCISCO

When we returned to Houston from Westby, Marlene busied herself opening additional wedding gifts and writing thank you cards while I poured over old State Board tests and information about them. We had to drive to Austin where the tests were given, and soon I was in the big hall where they were held, along with a number of other recent graduates. The test was pretty comprehensive, but I felt good about my answers; and so, after a good night's sleep, it was back to Houston to get packed for San Francisco. Marlene left most of our wedding gifts in Westby; therefore we were traveling light, with a four service dinner set, silverware, a few pots and pans, bedding, a floor lamp, clothing, and my saxophone.

The trip to San Francisco took three days, and we got there just before the July 1 start of the internship. We found a motel, and then went to the hospital for any help they could give us about a place to live. We were directed to an apartment house fairly close to the hospital. The apartment we were shown was rather dismal, filthy, and really appeared to be a dump. The rug in the front room was dirty and worn threadbare, and the furniture was nicked and marred. Marlene and I looked at each other. "What do you think?" I asked. "I couldn't stand to live in a place like this," she replied, so we struck out on our own. Luckily, we heard about a possible rental in a downstairs apartment on Rhode Island Street that had been rented to interns before.

We stopped there and met the landlords, Rudy and Marie Koenen, who were in the process of painting and getting it ready. They lived above. They told us that it would not be ready for a few more days but it was ours if we wanted it. It was perfect for us: I could walk down the hill and take a pedestrian bridge over a major thoroughfare to arrive at the emergency room entrance of San Francisco County Hospital. The apartment consisted of a bedroom with a couch that made out to a bed, a kitchen with a small breakfast table and chairs, and a bathroom with a shower. The bedroom windows looked out over a small steep backyard. There was another street below us, then the highway, and then San Francisco Hospital. Marlene started job hunting and it wasn't long before she had a good job at the Southern Pacific Hospital. Our rent was $150 a month, so money was a little tight, but we made out fine. We helped with the painting, and moved in the next day, before the paint was barely dry.

Rudy and Marie were wonderful landlords and were really like a couple of surrogate parents during our year in San Francisco. They showed us most of the sights of San Francisco, including Chinatown, Fisherman's Wharf, Golden Gate Bridge, Seal Rock, and several other places that tourists just don't go. They both spoke German, so I was able to brush up on my German grammar from college. Rudy had been a baker all his life until he retired, and then his hobby was photography. He still made some awfully good strudel with which he frequently blessed us. Marie was active in Eastern Star and seemed to know just about everybody. She could be considered one of San Francisco's "characters," but in a good sense of the word.

There was an orientation at the hospital on July 1 for the interns, and we got the bad news that they were three interns short. The schedule would place us on call two out of three nights and two out of three weekends. I was looking for a place to get a lot of experience so I obviously got my wish. In addition to my meager salary, I also got laundry and meals. The nights on call usually meant that we were up a good portion of the night, plus the full day of work, so every third night I tried to make up for the lack of sleep by being early to bed. That didn't leave much time to enjoy the sights of San Francisco.

When I was a medical student, we had to draw all the blood for the ward each morning and the interns at Jeff Davis got out of that duty. Here, it was reversed. The interns had that job and the medical students didn't get that "great experience." We also had to do a complete blood count and urinalysis on each of our patients which saved the lab a lot of time and expense. I had my own microscope that Elmer Schulze had given me, and I took it with me from service to service.

The wards accommodated about 30 patients, and the beds were lined around the room with an open space in the center to allow for the nurses' activity and medicine carts. Curtains separated each bed from the next, allowing very little privacy. All of the services were continually busy, and I usually had about six admissions a day plus 30 or 40 inpatients to care for. There was much to learn and I got along well with all the residents physicians except for one on the surgery rotation.

I had a burn patient and the resident had a strict bias to avoid any antibiotics for fear of developing resistant organisms. My patient developed a symptomatic urinary tract infection and her urine was loaded with bacilli. Besides the pain from her burns, she was miserable with urinary pain. I wanted to put her on sulfa to combat the infection which had the potential of spreading upward into her kidneys, but the resident was completely against treating it. When he left, I went against his orders and treated her anyway. He was furious and we went around and around about my countermanding his orders until an attending physician from the staff decided the argument in my favor. The resident never liked me after that.

There were a number of patients with end stage cirrhosis, and they presented with huge distended abdomens from the massive ascites. We would have to place a large trocar into their abdomen and drain out several liters of fluid in order to give them some comfort and better ability to eat and breathe. Since we had no long term alcoholic rehabilitation program, they were on a revolving door existence. We would keep them about two weeks, build up their nutrition and then dismiss them. About a month later we would see them back with the same problem until they finally died from either liver failure or hemorrhage from esophageal varices.

During my year at San Francisco County we had a severe outbreak of staph aureus infections. Almost all of the interns developed boils, and I was no exception. I had two large boils on my neck that were really a nuisance until they came to a head and drained. We could not go into surgery if we had any obvious boils, which reduced the number of interns available to scrub in surgery. Despite all of the measures to control the problem, nothing seemed to help, and wound infections were common in post- op patients. The epidemic finally just seemed to die out on its own after several months. I became ill with a cough, and when I ran a sputum specimen on myself, it was filled with staphylococcal bacteria. An X-ray showed a patch of pneumonia, so I ended up spending a few days in the isolation ward taking erythromycin until my fever broke and the pneumonia improved.

The obstetrical service was fairly busy, and since I had a lot of experience as a medical student with saddle block and forceps, I was given more latitude by the resident than some of the other interns. I got to assist on several C-sections and learn the technique of the procedure, but the residents were hungry for as much experience as possible, so interns were always just the assistant. However, they did let me do a few tubal ligations and incidental appendectomies as part of the total procedure.

Sometimes we had a little time off during the day, and the top floor of the hospital had a recreation room for the doctors. Some of us played bridge, and occasionally we would be short a player. We would call the operator and page Dr. Fourthbridge. I don't think the operator ever caught on.

The emergency room was always a place of unbelievable activity and interesting sights. I remember one of the street people who had a large chronic ulcer on his leg. When we got his trousers off, the wound was crawling with maggots, but surprisingly, the wound looked clean. The maggots had eaten all the necrotic, dead tissue away, and although this sounds pretty gross, it was a form of treatment that was used on purpose in days long past. The use of maggots has been revived in recent years for a few select cases. Trauma, broken bones, lacerations, and acute medical problems filled the area, and probably inspired the current TV programs about life in the ER.

The rotation on the TB service was rather interesting. We actually had the patients locked up, since many would have left before they were pronounced noncontagious. It was thought that if the infected lung could be put at rest with no movement, it could heal the cavities easier. Consequently, several procedures were tried. Creating an artificial pneumothorax was done but this had to be repeated about every two weeks as the air instilled into the chest to collapse the lung was absorbed. There was even a procedure to fill the chest cavity with ping pong balls to keep the lung from expanding. Creating a pneumoperitoneum (air instilled into the abdomen) was also done and repeated at weekly intervals, similar to what we do when we perform laparoscopic surgery. These barbaric procedures have long since been discontinued as we have developed better drugs to treat tuberculosis. I did get some additional surgical experience assisting with partial lung resections to remove badly diseased areas that would keep the patients contagious, and I did learn how to do a tracheotomy at that time. These were put in on a temporary basis in order to be able to suction out mucus and material that the patient was unable to cough up. This would prove valuable later.

When Marlene and I would occasionally get a night off together, we would go down to Market Street and eat supper at one of the "$1.09" steak houses. You could actually get a steak, salad, bread, and coffee for a dollar and nine cents. If you wanted a baked potato, it was another dollar. Rarely, we would treat ourselves to a more expensive dinner at Fisherman's Wharf. I remember one occasion that I really got "in the dog house." Marlene had bought some luscious blackberries, some small shortcakes, and some cream. She pinned a note on the refrigerator that said "eat all of it." When I got home from the hospital I saw the note, and being a good husband I took her at her word, and dutifully went back for a second and third helping until I had finished it all. Marlene came home when she got off her three to eleven shift, anticipating eating a helping of all three ingredients and there was nothing there. Evidently, we needed to work on our communication a little better. "Eat it all" and "Eat all of it" meant the same to me.

As the year progressed, I had to make plans as to how to do my postponed military obligation. Going in as an Army doctor did not promise as much hands on experience as I wanted, since most of the soldiers were healthy. Several of the interns were talking about the Indian Health branch of the Public Health Service. This made more sense to me, so I filled out the appropriate documents, got my physical, and got ready for an assignment when my year long internship finished. Finally, induction was held and I was to be assigned a post as Assistant Surgeon at White Earth Indian Hospital on the Chippewa reservation in White Earth, Minnesota. We had made several good friends during our stay in San Francisco, and it was like saying goodbye to our parents when we took our departure from Rudy and Marie. We did manage to visit them again several years later when we went back to California for my family practice residency. Now, it was off to the Land of Sky Blue Waters!

CHAPTER 11
INDIAN HEALTH SERVICE

As usual, we had very little time to get half way across the country from California to Minnesota. My internship ended on June 30, and I was supposed to be at my duty station in White Earth on July 2. We got started a little late, so our first night we stopped at Reno. We took in a few of the sights, but money was still tight and it would be a while before either of us got a paycheck. Fortunately, gasoline was still cheap in those days, averaging about forty-five cents a gallon. The next day we went through Salt Lake City and made it as far as Rawlins, Wyoming. From there we made it to Pierre, South Dakota, and the next day we found ourselves arriving at White Earth. As we saw the sign, we pulled into a dusty area where there was a small grocery store, and across the street, a flag pole and post office. I asked Marlene, "Where do you think the town is?" She replied with a smile, "I think you're in it."

We got directions to the hospital, which was a few streets away, none of which were paved. "This really looks like the boondocks to me," I said. I presented myself to the hospital nurses' station and introduced myself. The nurse on duty got in touch with the one remaining physician, Dr. Radke. Soon he was filling me in on the way the hospital was run. There were to be two physicians to staff the hospital, but the second physician, Dr. Roy Wittwer, would not be arriving for a few more days. Dr. Radke was anxious to wind up his affairs and leave, so that would leave me alone to staff the place for about a week. Just my luck, but I was getting used to that by now. Dr. Radke showed us the house that we were to occupy, and it was pretty old and drafty. There were also mice that flitted across the room occasionally, but we found that we would inherit a resident dog, "Smiley," who was an excellent mouse catcher.

61

He was old, and slightly arthritic. But, when a mouse appeared, he would forget about stiffness and pain, and act like a young dog again as he pounced on the mouse. He got his name from the rare quality in a dog of being able to curl his lips into a smile when you would call him or pet him. He proved to be a wonderful pet, but he did not like Chippewa Indians, because he had been abused when he was younger. This brings up an interesting story that I will relate in a later chapter.

The director of nurses was Miss Komove, a battle hardened lady, but a good nurse, from whom I learned a lot during my two years in the Indian Service. Clinic was held at the hospital on Monday, Wednesday, and Friday. On Tuesday and Thursday we had outreach clinic at Ponsford and Natawash, two smaller towns, about thirty-five miles from White Earth. Mornings were spent on rounds and emergencies. We had surgery once a week.

The lab was pretty primitive, and the technician was a girl who had taken one of the short lab courses lasting about a year or less. No one had used the colorimeter recently, so blood chemistries were not being done. There was no functioning incubator, so no cultures could be performed. I was back in my element again, and it was not long before we had standardized the colorimeter for some basic chemistries. I ordered some petri dishes and culture media powder to use for bacterial culture plates. Soon we began to look like a real lab. Pregnancy tests were not available, but then an interesting event happened.

First, I must tell you about the evolution of pregnancy tests. The first test devised was the rabbit test. In this test, a rabbit is injected with urine from a pregnant woman. Forty- eight hours later the rabbit is sacrificed and the ovaries are examined. If the woman was pregnant, the rabbit's ovaries would show hemorrhages from ovulation due to the hormones in the woman's urine. The next advance in pregnancy testing was the frog test. In this test, five milliliters of a patient's morning urine is injected under the loose skin of a male frog. Four hours later the frog is grabbed, and in the process, he will usually squirt urine, which is directed toward a large glass slide if the technician is skillful and quick. Under the microscope, one will see rosettes of sperm if the urine contains the hormones of pregnancy.

And now to the story. I was walking around the back part of our lawn one evening when I heard, "Croak, Croak, Croak." I began to look closely toward the area of the sounds, and to my surprise I saw several green and yellow spotted frogs. They were Rana Pipiens (northern leopard frogs), the same kind that we used in the pregnancy tests and had to order from New York by special delivery in boxes filled with moss. They were jumping around in the backyard. I caught several, and put them in a card board box prior to placing them in the refrigerator bin to keep them in hibernation, along with some local moss from the oak trees. "Now that is fine," you are probably saying, "but if you are not a frog, how in the world do you tell the males from the females?" Well, actually it is quite simple. The males have a much more muscular thumb, used for grasping the females, which is a lot different from the delicate hand and thumb of the female. So now our lab had an up to date pregnancy test without having to order special delivery.

Dr. Wittwer arrived about a week into the month and we rapidly got acquainted. His house was next to ours and he was to be the medical officer in charge. He had just finished the surgical year of his family practice residency at Sacramento, California, and was senior to me in experience. That was nice, because I had someone to mentor me in surgical procedures done by family doctors. Roy had done a lot of orthopedics during that year also. We certainly would have a lot of broken bones to treat.

We did have a surgeon, Dr. Finklestein, from Bemidji, Minnesota, who was doing mostly administration for the Indian Service. He was happy to come down on surgical days to do procedures and teach. Miss Komove did our anesthesia, mostly ether, but some pentathol with curare. I won't say our operating room was antiquated, but we did have one nurse assigned to swat flies during the procedures. Minnesota is a state filled with insects in the summer, and even though we had screened windows in the hospital, including the operating room, it was impossible to keep them out. Fortunately, we had practically no wound infections as we had seen in the big city hospitals.

Tonsillectomies were done without intubation, which we would never consider now, because of the chance of aspirating blood into the lungs during the procedure. However, if the assistant was attentive and suctioned quickly and carefully, especially with the patient in the head down position, we never had a problem. I learned to do a fairly respectable tonsillectomy, but I became more skilled with this procedure during my residency. A family doctor, who was doing the anesthesia, pointed out a few little tricks that made the procedure much less bloody and considerably quicker. More later.

Roy's wife was named Deedee, and they had a three year old son named Mark. Deedee was a brunette, but Mark was a towheaded blond, and sort of resembled my blond wife. Frequently, Marlene, Deedee and Mark would make a trip to Detroit Lakes to shop. Deedee felt that it was best to let young children explore their surroundings and have very little restraint. Consequently, she did not supervise him when he was in the grocery store. The clerks would turn to my wife when Mark got off limits and say, "Your kid is behind the counter and into the cakes." Once Mark actually climbed up and fell into the pickle barrel. Marlene got the blame again.

Roy was a bow hunter and introduced me to the sport. We set up targets made of hay bales behind our houses and had a good practice range. Then I learned how to make bow strings and fletch arrows. Marlene and I picked out some recurve bows in the now defunct Herter's catalog. Marlene got a thirty-six pound target bow and I got a slightly heavier hunting bow. We went to archery shoots occasionally, where a course was laid out with fourteen targets at various distances varying from twenty feet to eighty yards. We would shoot four arrows at the bull's-eye targets for the first round, and four at animal targets for the second. I never got a deer with a bow while in Minnesota, but I bagged several, including an elk, when I moved to Montana.

Our first experience with skiing was in Minnesota. There was a small hill outside of Detroit Lakes, and an enterprising farmer had fashioned a rope tow attached to a tractor wheel to pull the skiers up the hill. It was quite a job to hold on to the rope and be pulled up the hill with your skis following the deep ruts from other skiers. Then the trick of snowplowing down the hill for us novices proved quite a task. When you fall down as a novice, even the job of getting up on skis is hard to do, and we spent a lot of time doing that. Oh well, the longest journey starts with the first small step.

Minnesota is a land of many small lakes, all filled with Northern Pike, Walleyes, and perch. Roy had a canoe and we managed to get into a few of the small lakes that had no access by car. We had to carry his canoe about a quarter of a mile, and then sort of wade through the marsh grass and cattails in order to launch it. It was worth the effort, and we would have the lake all to ourselves, where very little fishing had been done. We used Daredevil red and white lures on spinning rods and we would get a strike on almost every cast. Most were small Northern Pike, but every few casts we would latch onto a 24 inch fish and have quite a fight on our hands. Because Northern Pike are filled with small bones, it takes a larger one that can be filleted to make it worthwhile to save for eating. They are among the tastiest of fish. When my parents came to visit us, and I took my father fishing, he had a hard time throwing back those 12 inch pike in order to get a larger one. I finally convinced him that because they were so plentiful, with a little patience, a bigger one would find its way onto his hook.

We had a lake behind the hospital that was a spot that the northern ducks would use in their flights south during their migration. During hunting season, we would go down to the lake after work to shoot our limit. If we were on call for the outpatient clinic, it posed a problem for us. We did not have walkie-talkies or radios with which to communicate with the hospital, so we worked out a system. If an outpatient came in after hours, but before sunset, while we were still hunting, the nurse would go outside to one of the staff cars and honk the horn according to a prearranged signal. It worked fine and we got in a little extra hunting for the effort.

The lakes that we fished in the summer gave us another excellent outdoor sport in the winter, namely, ice skating. The ice would freeze to several feet thick so that breaking through was not a worry. We could take our snow shovels along and clear some nice runs if there was snow piled up, but many times there were long stretches of bare ice that offered unimpeded skating for hundreds of yards. There were occasional cracks in the ice that could catch our skates and send us tumbling if we were not careful to plan our path in advance. It was very exhilarating to skate along these bare stretches of ice. One could feel like Hans Brinker in Holland as he skated the long frozen waterways in the book, "Hans Brinker and the Silver Skates." Ice fishing was also a fun winter sport that I did on occasions.

Winters could get cold with a lot of snow. I remember an incident when we sent home a mother and newborn. The mother was having trouble nursing and couldn't get her milk flowing so we sent her home with some bottles, nipples, and a small amount of formula until she could get back in for a checkup a few days later. Then a terrible snow storm hit and the snow piled up so that it was impossible to get around even on the main roads. Travel was at a standstill, and this family really lived back in the "boonies." We sort of forgot about their plight until we saw the mother with her well fed plump baby four weeks later. I noticed that her breasts had returned to normal and that she was not nursing. "What were you able to feed your baby for the weeks when you couldn't get out to come to the clinic for more formula?" I asked. "Rabbit soup," the mother replied. Her husband had been able to shoot enough rabbits to keep them in food, and she had cooked the rabbit meat until it became gruel. She had an apple tree behind her house and they had laid in a supply of apples in the root cellar, and also a supply of potatoes. She cooked up the apples to make apple sauce and added that to the mixture in addition to some well boiled and mashed potatoes for additional calories. After thinning it with water it made a fairly decent formula, and the baby could take it through a slightly enlarged hole in the nipple. Necessity is the mother of invention!

During my time at White Earth, I became well-liked by the Indians. During one of their powwows, I was adopted into the tribe. That was quite an honor, since I was the first Indian Health Service doctor to be adopted. They gave me the name "Mushkekee Oneenee," which means medicine man in Chippewa. Naturally, I had to dance around the circle and that made quite a sight with me throwing my head up and down and skipping along to the rhythm of the drums.

The old chief (I forget his name) had a huge rhinophyma, which is a large bulbous nose due to proliferation of connective tissue and oil gland enlargement from years of drinking and probably some hereditary predisposition. Although he was in his eighties, he wanted it fixed, since it hung over into his coffee cup when he tried to drink coffee. His nose even had Jimmy Durante's trumped in size.

It looked like it would be quite an undertaking, so I referred him to the plastic surgery department at the medical school in Minneapolis. For some reason, they declined to operate on him due to his age or some other cause, so he was back to see me, begging for some help. "Doc, can't you do something about this? They told me they couldn't help me when I went to the University," he said.

I guess I was too young to realize all the things that could possibly go wrong, but I said that I would give it a try. I decided to work on one side at a time and see how the healing went instead of trying to reduce the size of his nose in one sitting. I used local anesthesia and started on the left side first, making an incision, cutting a large chunk of tissue away and then shaping it so I could close the incision without too much tension. It was fairly bloody, but I could control the bleeders with electrocoagulation. It looked pretty good when I finished and when he returned in about ten days it had healed beautifully. I took courage in this, and did the other side in the same fashion. I had reduced the size considerably on the sides but the tip still hung over in front, so with the third procedure I cut a large transverse ellipse out, undermined it toward the tip and then pulled it up and back to close the defect. This lifted and shortened his nose. When it healed, he was pleased as punch, and could drink coffee without burning his nose. I carried a picture of him before and after in my wallet for years to show off my first plastic surgery.

Occasionally we made calls with the Public Health Nurse to some of the homes. I really had my eyes opened to some pretty wretched living conditions. The conditions could have been markedly improved if some of those families had taken a little more pride in their surroundings by simple measures to fix up and clean their surroundings a bit. I remember one family that needed a bed and mattress. One was given to them. It laid outside for weeks in the rain and weather because the man of the house said his back was bad and he couldn't carry it inside.

One mystery was cleared up during a visit that we made about lunch time, regarding one of our pharmacy drugs, syrup of White Pine, a cough preparation. The family was having pancakes, and guess what they were using to top their pancakes? Syrup of White Pine. Needless to say, we were a little more careful with our prescribing in the future.

67

Since gallbladder disease was quite prevalent among the Indians, I was getting a great deal of experience taking out gallbladders. Roy and I decided that we didn't have to call Dr. Finklestein for every gallbladder and we were now on our own for the majority of the procedures. We had a regional meeting for the Aberdeen region of Indian Health and each of the hospitals were supposed to enter a project.

We decided to make a movie of the technique of cholecystectomy. We got someone from the hospital with a 16 mm camera to photograph one of our easier cholecystectomies. It turned out great and we got some favorable comments for our work. I was getting some really great experience in the broad range of general practice at White Earth.

My two years in the Indian Health Service were soon ending.

I knew that there were still areas in which I needed to improve, so I began looking at Family Practice residencies. Roy told me about several in California. I applied for a position at Monterey County Hospital in Salinas, California, and I was accepted. I knew that I wanted to eventually practice in Montana, the "Big Sky Country," so Marlene and I decided to use some of our vacation time to look around the state. Marlene's father, Tony, was a pilot and flew a Cessna that he used in conjunction with his implement business. He agreed to fly us around the state to check out several of the towns.

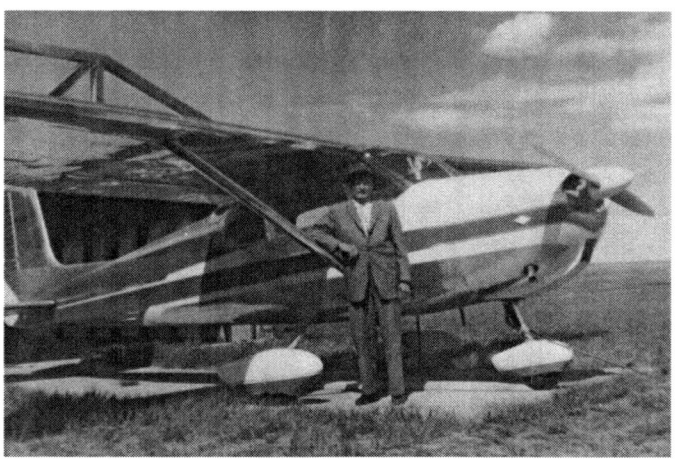

Tony and his airplane.

Since I had really wanted to be in western Montana, we first flew to Kalispell to look over that area. I still looked somewhat young for my age of 29, and I routinely got carded when we would order alcoholic beverages. We went uptown to one of the hotels in Kalispell and signed in. The man at the desk turned to the bell hop and said, "Take the bags up to the rooms for the man, the woman, and the boy." Marlene hasn't lived that down yet.

From Kalispell we went to Polson, Big Fork, Hamilton, and Lewistown. Most of the doctors that we met were cordial, but I got the impression that they didn't want anyone invading their turf. I was encouraged to get more training before deciding where to practice. One of the doctors in Lewistown, however, told me that Hardin really needed a doctor, and that I should check it out.

Our next scheduled stop was Miles City, since I was not really that interested in the flat scenery around Hardin. As we flew over it, Tony, Marlene's father, said, "Maybe we should stop and give Hardin a look since I am a little low on gas." We swung the plane around and landed at the small airport just next to the end of Center Avenue, which was the main street. "Why don't we walk down a few blocks and stretch our legs and get a cup of coffee," Tony said.

We ended up at the Lobby Cafe, and as we were seated, the waitress asked us where we were from. Tony said, "This is my son-in-law, a doctor, and he is looking for a place to practice." Before we had finished our first cup of coffee, we were surrounded by one of the county commissioners, Carey Mabe, the clerk of court, Harry Cox, and the president of the Big Horn Bank, Leroy (Wally) Wallin. They told me that they were really desperate for a physician because one was leaving for a radiology residency and the other was in poor health. They said that the building of the Yellowtail Dam was in progress and there were many workers adding to the population of Big Horn County.

They extolled the beauty of the Big Horn River and all of the hunting and fishing in the surrounding area, in addition to the closeness of Billings for shopping and cultural events. There would be no shortage of patients, and, before the second cup of coffee, I had agreed to come to Hardin when I finished the one year rotating residency at Monterey County Hospital.

There was supposed to be a second physician recruited so that the load would not be overwhelming. There was also talk of building a clinic building. With that out of the way, we skipped Miles City and flew back to Westby for the rest of the short vacation. Then it was back to White Earth for the last month of my tour of duty.

I found out that in the coming year, the Indian Health Service was planning to close White Earth for inpatient care, and transfer those patients to Detroit Lakes under the contract care program. The hospital was getting a little too antiquated for modern day inpatient medicine. I managed to get a lot of inpatient experience that the doctors following me would miss out on. I had some offers to go into practice at a clinic in Detroit Lakes, but I knew that I was still a little weak in a few aspects of family practice, especially ENT. A year of rotating Family Practice residency would be helpful in strengthening those areas.

The end of June was arriving and we began preparing to leave. We hired a man with a truck to haul our small amount of accumulated furniture, TV, and other stuff to Salinas, California. Finally, the day arrived, and we began our journey across the country in our newly acquired Rambler station wagon along with Smiley, our dog, who we could not bear to leave behind for a new owner.

It was back toward the Pacific Ocean again.

CHAPTER 12
SALINAS

Our trip back to California started along the same route we had taken on our arrival to Minnesota, but when we arrived in Belle Fourche, somehow we made a wrong turn. After driving about forty miles, we noticed that the country looked more desolate than we had remembered. I noticed that according to the sun, we were traveling northwest instead of southwest. Sure enough, we were headed toward Broadus, Montana. That accounted for the desolate look, so we had to backtrack. Soon we were again on our planned route. From Cheyenne, Wyoming, we went directly west to Salt Lake City, and then to Ely, Nevada. We decided to visit Yosemite National Park, which provided some spectacular scenery along the way. Finally, we arrived in Salinas and found our way to Monterey County Hospital. We met with Dr. Whitworth, the medical director, and then began house hunting. We found a moderately priced rental on the outskirts of Salinas, about a fifteen minute drive to the hospital. It was just on the edge of the artichoke and onion fields. We had a fair sized back and front yard which was fenced for our dog, Smiley. There was even room to set up some hay bales in the back yard for archery targets.

All of the new residents met with Dr. Whitworth, the medical director. We found out that we would be on first call every third night, and second call, which usually didn't keep us up, every fourth night. We did have to sleep at the hospital, however, on those nights. This residency rotated through most of the specialties over a year's duration, and then repeated again the second year. I had only planned to take a one year program. We had no interns or students, but we did have attending staff in all the specialties. Two of the residents were taking their second yea:, and seven of us were taking our first year. It was a diverse group, and we all got along well. The oldest was J. P. O'Halloren, a little older than the rest of us and with a family of seven children. I think he had been in practice a few years and just wanted to brush up a little. He had a petite little wife who certainly didn't look bedraggled for having seven children. I remember that he was on the phone with his stock broker much of the time, but most of the rest of us didn't know anything about stocks, nor did we have any money to invest anyway.

I knew that I wanted to spend time with the ENT doctors, since I didn't want to be referring out cases, that with a little extra training, I could handle. I had not fixed any broken noses and needed to know how to properly anesthetize a nose with local anesthetic and then reduce the fracture. We had an excellent ENT attending physician who taught me how to do that in a short time. We were allowed to do the tonsillectomies on the service and I got to do quite a few. Once when I was in the process of a slightly difficult one, the anesthetist, who was also a family doctor, said, "Let me show you how to make that a little easier." He showed me how to put a little more forward traction on the tonsil with the tonsil tenaculum, and then gently scoop under it in a forward sweeping motion. It separated beautifully from the posterior tonsillar fossa a lot easier than I had ever gotten it to do before. It's amazing that when you think you know how to do something pretty well, and then are shown how to improve your technique, how much easier things get. I have taught young doctors just learning to do tonsillectomies the same procedure since that time with good results. I learned how to pack a nose properly for nosebleed, and also how to use the inflatable balloons for the posterior bleeders. I had not had to treat any nosebleeds as an intern and really not many while in the Indian Service. The ENT rotation gave me added confidence in those areas.

J.P. O'Halloren and I were on the surgical service together. I made it a point to get the attending surgeon to let me do the cases that would be the ones I would hopefully be doing once I got into private practice. They were, for the most part, accommodative. That gave me additional experience to follow up my White Earth surgical procedures in hernias, appendectomies, and gallbladders. I also developed a better knowledge of bowel anastomosis, and resection. I did skin grafts and dermatologic procedures for skin cancers to round out my rotation.

Once, J.P. and I were assisting the neurosurgeon with the removal of a meningioma. This was my first time assisting in opening a skull down to the meninges of the brain. Bleeding had to be controlled, and the tumor exposed. It then had to be removed, and the piece of skull replaced, the fascia and temporal muscle sutured over it, and the skin closed. Well, the meningioma was removed, and everything went OK for a few hours, and then the patient started to go bad due to some bleeding that had evidently not been well controlled inside the skull. We called the neurosurgeon to report the problem, expecting him to rush back the thirty miles from Carmel and open the patient's head again. He said, "You boys know how to do that now, so I'm going to let you handle it." We were more than a little scared, but we carefully took out the sutures, wires, and the piece of skull, found the bleeder after cleaning out the clots, and then closed up the wound again. The patient made an uneventful recovery.

Once, when I was observing a bronchoscopy, the surgeon doing the procedure noted a suspicious lump at the junction of two of the bronchi. Unfortunately, the lump was being pushed up by an anomalous large artery. When his biopsy forceps bit into the area, it opened up this artery and the blood came spurting out, totally preventing us from any sort of rescue. The patient bled out before anyone could even set up a surgical room. That was my first experience with a real surgical catastrophe. It left a lasting impression as to how a relatively minor procedure can suddenly result in an unexpected death, proving that all things don't always go as planned.

On the obstetrical service I added another 50 deliveries to my list, and a couple more C-sections. There were a few more toxemias of pregnancy treated and a number of tubal ligations performed post delivery. I helped with bladder repairs and hysterectomies enough to feel secure doing them without supervision, as I knew that would probably be the case.

Marlene was about three months pregnant when we arrived in Salinas, but was her usual bundle of energy. She got a job at one of the local hospitals until she was about seven months along. All of the residents had the chief of the obstetrical service, Dr. Klinefelter, for their wives' doctor, and most seemed to be or would soon be pregnant during that year. Marlene's prenatal course was uneventful except that she went several weeks overdue. When she finally went into labor, it was very prolonged. Husbands were not really welcomed in the delivery suite in those years, and were relegated to the waiting room or just told to stay out of the way until the baby was born.

I was able to spend a little time with Marlene, and noted that she just didn't seem to be progressing normally. I was not really going to start questioning the chief of the service about this, however, as one would probably do today. I was sent back to the county hospital to do three surgeries that I had on my schedule for that day, and when I returned, not much had changed. She was continually sedated with meperidine, but made no progress. It would be obvious today that when a woman is overdue by several weeks and then has a labor that is not progressing, she is probably occiput posterior and the baby can't proceed down the birth canal in the usual fashion. She will need some help either by a forceps rotation or a C-section.

They just kept sedating Marlene and telling her to push. Finally after her third trip into the delivery room and then a return trip to the labor room, she grabbed onto the side rails and said, "I'm not leaving." Finally Dr. Klinefelter came, and discovered that she was occiput posterior. He managed to apply forceps, turn the baby, and deliver her. Today, Marlene would probably have had a C-section for postmaturity, and certainly would not have been subjected to about thirty-six hours of hard labor. We were lucky that there was no damage to our daughter, Lois.

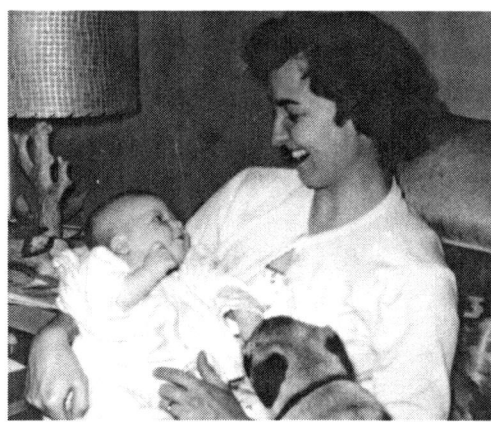

Marlene with baby Lois

And now, back to the story about our dog, Smiley. As I said, he had been abused on the reservation by some of the Chippewa Indians, and he really hated them. We lived on the outskirts of Salinas by the vegetable fields that were tended by the Mexican workers. They walked by our place continuously without causing Smiley to bark or growl at them. One day, there was a knock at our front door, and Smiley went ballistic. The fur rose on his back and he began growling and barking and tearing at the door. "What's wrong with you Smiley?" Marlene said. She held him by the collar and opened the door, and guess what? There was an Indian at the door who had stopped by and wondered if she could fix him a sandwich or provide him with something to eat. He told her that he was from Minnesota and had recently come to California. Since he was from Minnesota, he was naturally a Chippewa. Smiley had Chippewas hard wired into his memory. Marlene fixed him a sandwich and he was on his way.

The coast of California around Monterey is really beautiful with its white sand beaches and blue water. We would frequently take a scenic drive along that stretch of highway known as the "Seventeen Mile Drive." Sometimes we would wander down the beach and dig up a bag of clams for a meal when we returned to Salinas. Once at low tide, we went out to an exposed oyster outcropping, and broke off some of the oysters to take back home to fry and have on the half shell. For crabbing, it was possible to wade out into the surf until the water was about waist deep and drive a stake into the sandy bottom. A cord was then attached to it and baited with a chunk of stew meat. When a crab had been attracted to it, the cord could be slowly pulled up and a crab net slipped under the crab. With a few successful attempts, we would have enough crabs for a meal.

We made one trip back to San Francisco to see Rudy and Marie, and we spent the weekend with them. There was a German freighter in the harbor, and Marie knew the captain. We were invited on board for lunch and had a wonderful authentic German meal. We visited Chinatown and saw one of the places where fortune cookies were made. They gave us a bag of the rejects that didn't turn out just right, but they tasted just as good anyway. Rudy seldom went to church, although Marie attended Catholic Mass regularly. He said the last time he went, there was a pretty severe earthquake, and that was telling him something. We drove back to Salinas after a wonderful weekend, but unfortunately, never got to see them again. Rudy had a fatal heart attack shortly afterward, and a year later Marie began to develop rapidly progressing Alzheimer's disease and had to be placed in a nursing home.

We were in a mild earthquake while in Salinas, although the epicenter was some distance away. The bed began to shake and it felt like someone was under our bed and trying to get out. We finally realized what was happening, and got up to check on things. Aside from a few cabinet doors being knocked open and some canned goods rolling out, no real damage was done. It was a bit scary, however, and that is as close as I hope to get to a real earthquake.

Since my residency was drawing to a close, I had to apply for a Montana license to practice medicine. I had used my Texas license to get reciprocity for California and could do the same for Montana. I had to have a personal interview with the Montana Board of Medical Examiners first. It was a slightly difficult task to get from Salinas to Helena Montana and then back without losing significant time in travel and connections. Tony and his airplane proved to be the solution. He was glad to fly out to Salinas for a visit, take me to Helena and back, and have a good excuse to do some flying to new places at the same time. We had a good trip, but when I met with the Board of Medical Examiners, I was a little disappointed. The interview consisted of, "You say you're currently in Salinas? That's where they raise all those artichokes, isn't it? Well, good to have you in Montana. We need more doctors in small towns here." I guess the purpose of the interview was to make sure I didn't have two heads or a third eye in the middle of my forehead.

The residency was ending, so we again hired a truck to ship our belongings to Hardin, and then we began our trip to eastern Montana. The truck would take about two weeks to bring our furniture. The plan was to find a place to live, and then for Marlene and Lois to go to Westby until the furniture and "stuff" arrived. We were on our way back to the Big Sky County!

CHAPTER 13
HARDIN

We arrived in Hardin and pulled into the Lariat Motel, tired and a little apprehensive about all the things that were necessary in order to start a practice. It is easy to go to work for someone else when everything is there from the start, including your salary. No one had done anything about building a clinic building, and there was no definite news about a second doctor to replace Dr. Gilcrest, who had left for a radiology residency several months previously. That night, we lay awake wondering where to start. Marlene said, "Let's not stay. We can go back to the Park and work for the summer there, and then plan what we should do." It was tempting, but the town was so short of medical care that I just could not do it. Since I had made sort of a commitment, I felt we should stay and give it a chance. Dr. McFarland was still there, but his health was not good, and most of the patients were making the long trip to Billings on the narrow two lane highway 87. The hospital really needed to have medical care stay in Hardin if it was to survive.

The next morning I met with Mr. Wallin at the bank, and found that borrowing money to get started was not a problem. The hospital administrator was named Chuck Halls, and he was very good in helping me make plans for my practice. Chuck had joined the Navy at seventeen, and spent twenty years as a corpsman. He then retired from the Navy, and went to work for Lutheran Homes and Hospitals, which was the management company for the Hardin hospital. He did a lot more than the hospital administrators do today. Besides the administrative duties, he doubled as the director of nurses, filled in as part time lab and x-ray technician, took care of the walking blood bank, and ended up being my surgical assistant. Of course, that was a different day and time, and rules and regulations were not so burdensome in that era. Everyone concentrated on patient care, and were not worrying about being politically correct. Common sense ruled in those days.

The next thing on my agenda was to find space to open my practice. Since there was no clinic building, we found three adjacent rooms in the Kronmiller building which had the potential to work, although they were far from ideal. The first room would serve as the waiting room, and the second adjacent room could be partitioned into two examination rooms with a small hall leading to the third room, which would be for the charts, lab, medical supplies, refrigerator and a small desk for me. We hired a carpenter to make the necessary changes, and he went to work. The next thing on the agenda was to get the required medical equipment for the practice. Mr. Halls put me in touch with Northwest Surgical Supply and I was off to Billings. The people at Northwest Surgical Supply were very helpful, and I purchased two used exam tables, stools, goose necked lamps, and a supply cabinet. We bought a small metal desk and chair for me, a centrifuge and sterilizer, and then a few chairs for the waiting room. We used the couch that we had in our possession from our days at White Earth, to provide a little more seating in the waiting room.

We next rented an apartment from Joe and Jean Koebbe, but since our furniture had not yet arrived, Marlene, Lois, and our new Pug dog Spike, that we had purchased in Salinas, went back to Westby to await its arrival. I would be sleeping on the floor of our apartment in my bedroll with the phone by my side for those first two weeks, and it was ringing off the wall, (or more correctly, off the floor). Since the office was not ready at that time, I was practicing out of the hospital, using a patient room, and making house calls. I hired a bookkeeper to come in to tally up the records at the end of the day. When our furniture arrived and the office renovation was mostly completed, Marlene returned from Westby, and took over the duties as my nurse. By this time, she was pregnant with our second child, Marc, and I needed to be looking for a nurse so Marlene could be home with Lois. I hired Dorine Morse, who was a devoted and wonderful nurse for the thirty years that she worked for me before she and her husband moved to Billing. Dorine did more than just be in charge of the nursing at the clinic. When we were swamped she would triage the patients, sew up some of the lacerations, put on casts, and handle some of the more minor problems. She was a nurse practitioner before there were nurse practitioners.

We were swamped with patients from the start, and it was a relief when the remodeling was completed and we could move into our quarters at the Kronmiller building. Besides the patients from Hardin and the surrounding areas, the 3000 new inhabitants from Fort Smith needed for the building of Yellowtail Dam, were added to the mix. They were quite happy not to have to travel the forty seven miles from Fort Smith to Hardin, and then another fifty miles to get medical care in Billings. Office calls were four dollars for the initial visit and three dollars for a revisit for the same problem.

There were a lot of pregnant women also, and I believe I had 110 deliveries the first year in Hardin. There was no Medicaid for indigent patients in those days, so the county was responsible for their care. I negotiated a contract with the county, for which I received $450 a month for all of the patients that I believed fell within my expertise. It was very simple. They just came in and got care and there were no forms to fill out, and no reports to submit. That care included deliveries and any surgery that I could handle. When I think back, they really got a good deal, but I was happy, both for the guaranteed check and the chance to establish myself.

A few weeks after I arrived, our first real emergency occurred. A patient, Donna, who had been receiving her obstetrical care in Billings up to that point, presented to the hospital with major hemorrhaging. She was pale, going into shock, and we had to act quickly if we were going to save her life. She had what is known as placenta abruptio. It occurs when the placenta prematurely separates from the uterus. Small separations can be treated conservatively with bed rest and fluids, but a major bleed like she had required immediate transfusion and a C-section. When the placenta separates, not only does the mother lose a lot of blood, but the baby is deprived of the oxygen and nutrients that would cross that area of the placenta. Well, we had no blood stored in the lab refrigerator, no anesthetist, no pediatrician, and no second assistant doctor to help, so I was on my own,

The ambulance was just a station wagon, and that made it difficult to administer blood or fluids, due to its low ceiling. Besides, there was no place to hang a bottle of blood. We did have a walking blood bank with a few dozen names, so within a few minutes we had two donors lying on the table giving a pint of blood each. Mr. Halls cross matched the blood while one of the nurses was preparing the surgery room, since the way my patient was bleeding there was no chance to transfer her to her doctor in Billings. "Am I going to die?" she asked me in a weak voice. "No, we'll get you through this," I replied. "We just have to work fast." I found the spinal anesthetic tray and the pontacaine that I used for saddle blocks, and as soon as the blood was going, I gave her a spinal anesthetic, and instructed one of the nurses to administer oxygen and monitor her blood pressure. Chuck Halls had assisted in surgery before, as a Navy corpsman, so, with one other nurse to circulate, we began the emergency C-section. We still had to act quickly, and this was my first C-section alone with no other doctors and anesthetist to share the responsibility. I made a midline incision, quickly opened the abdomen, packed the bowel away from the uterus and then reflected the bladder flap downward on the lower part of the uterus. I made a transverse incision in the uterus, spread the incision laterally with my fingers, and reached in to dislodge the baby's head as the blood was pouring out. I delivered the baby, who thankfully started to cry, and I gave her to the nurse. I told my nurse who was handling the oxygen to administer pitocin to help the uterus clamp down and cut off the bleeding. I separated the placenta and removed it, and things now settled down to a more manageable state. Mr. Halls assisted me in closing up the incision in the uterus and then the abdominal wall. Hardin had witnessed its first C-section since the new hospital had been built. Mother and baby were stable. I leaned over the drape and said to Donna, the mother, "I told you that you would be all right." I was able to report this to the relatives and father who were waiting anxiously in the waiting room. "Are these the kind of emergencies that I am going to be faced with in the future?" I thought to myself.

CHAPTER 14
LADIES OF THE NIGHT

Nature abhors a vacuum, which was evident in the gold camps of the old West, where there was a surplus of young healthy men and a paucity of single women. This led to a thriving business of prostitution. Such was the case when Yellowtail Dam was being constructed at Fort Smith, Montana, which is forty-seven miles south of Hardin. It wasn't long after the start of the project when an enterprising Madam opened the P.M. Ranch, otherwise known as the "Bunkhouse." It was on the order of a motel and contained four "units" where the "girls" plied their trade. The Madam employed about four "girls." They would come to my office for checkups every two week for a pelvic exam, blood test for syphilis, and cultures to check for gonorrhea. It was not difficult to tell who they were when they were either sitting in the waiting room or walking down the street. Their makeup was heavy and their clothes were pretty flashy and provocative. After their exam, they would head to the drug store to buy cosmetics and sundries, and shop at the local dress shop.

Once, Marlene and I were walking down Center Avenue on a Thursday afternoon, which was their day to come to Hardin. As we passed one of the "girls," she said, "Hello, Dr. Whiting." "Who was that?" asked Marlene. "Just someone I know professionally," I said. "Yours or hers?" Marlene inquired.

It took about a year, but finally several of the pastors of our thirteen churches (we also had thirteen bars) brought enough pressure and complaints to the Sheriff so that he was forced to act. Roy Riley and his deputies raided the "Bunkhouse" and hauled   the girls off to jail.

They posted bond, left town, and the P.M. Ranch was officially closed for good.

Bob Wilson, County Attorney, was questioning one of the girls, whom he recognized as living in Ronan during his high school years. He had an older friend, a bomber pilot during WWII, who had returned to Ronan after the war with a new wife from New Orleans. She was quite a beauty. She had a beautiful southern drawl and a friendly manner. Bob lost track of them when he went away to college, but found out later that they had divorced and the wife's story was a tragic one of alcoholism, drugs, loss of custody of her children, and finally a slide into prostitution. When he questioned her, using her first name by which she was known in Ronan, she looked at him and said, "Are you Bob Wilson?" Bob offered her all the help that he could to get her out of the trade and into rehabilitation. Although she was grateful, she turned him down.

There is still a question about how we legislate morality. There was never any trouble from their activities, and they were free of any communicable disease as far as their medical exams were concerned. If we have to have prostitution, it is probably best done in a controlled environment, rather than have "streetwalkers."

This leads me into the next topic of venereal diseases. The four that I want to talk about are syphilis, gonorrhea, venereal warts, and chlamydia. In the 1960s, Herpes and HIV were not a concern.

Syphilis has been written about since at least the fifteenth century. Many European countries blame each other for its origin, such as the French disease, the Venetian, or Spanish affliction.

Voltaire wrote in one of his works that the first gift of the Spaniard to the New World was syphilis. This has been disputed, however, since the first major epidemic of syphilis occurred just after Columbus's sailors returned from the New World, indicating that they may have brought it back with them to infect Europe. Its origin still remains a question.

Early treatment involved the use of heavy metal compounds, especially mercury, which was extremely toxic. Infected people were placed in a type of barrel with just their head exposed and then the body was fumigated. Various compounds of mercury, antimony and arsenic were also ingested and applied to the skin in an effort to treat the disease. It has been said that "A night in the arms of Venus leads to a year in the clutches of Mercury."

It was not until 1905 that the spirochete of syphilis was identified by Paul Erlich. His compound, Salversan 606, was proved to cure the disease. Since it was made from arsenic, it was very toxic and the treatment was prolonged with occasional relapses. Finally, the advent of penicillin proved to be an effective and safe treatment.

Syphilis starts with a painless ulcer on the genitalia, associated with local lymph gland swelling and low grade fever. I had done microscopy on these lesions when I worked at Schulze's lab. A special darkfield condenser is attached to the microscope and the spirochetes can be seen as shimmering corkscrews against a dark background.

After a few weeks, the ulcer heals and secondary syphilis appears, consisting of a generalized skin rash which is very contagious with the spirochetes being present in the skin lesions. This phase can last for weeks, and can attack various organs of the body mimicking a number of other diseases. It has been said that he who knows syphilis well knows the history of medicine.

Finally, tertiary syphilis develops, attacking the heart, nervous system, brain, and vital organs, eventually causing death. Several people of note in history that were afflicted with syphilis were King Charles VIII, Ivan the Terrible, Franz Schubert, Paul Gauguin, Edouard Manet, Scott Joplin, and Al Capone.

Gonorrhea has been described for about as long as syphilis has been around, but it was not really identified as a separate disease until about the mid 1500s. It did not carry the same fatal consequences as syphilis, but still could wreck havoc with a woman's reproductive organs, and cause severe urethral problems in the male. A more common name for gonorrhea was the "Clap." This term may have come from the French word Clapier which means "brothel." However, a notorious eighteenth century Madam, by the name of Margaret Clap may also be the originator of the name.

Early treatment in the male consisted of irrigations of the urethra with various solutions of heavy metal salts but the best one of these seemed to be a dilute silver nitrate solution. Despite this, urethral strictures occurred which required dilations of the urethra to allow the bladder to empty.

When I was a medical student, a large part of the urology clinic was taken up with dilation procedures using progressively larger curved metal tubes called sounds. Occasionally, the stricture was so severe that a slightly flexible tiny tube was required to find the narrowed urethral tract into the bladder and then a stiff catheter was screwed onto the end and forced through the narrowed stricture in the urethra to break up the scar tissue, and allow sounds to then be passed to open a sufficiently large enough opening to allow the bladder to drain.

Penicillin, of course, brought a dramatic change in the treatment of this disease. Now the bacteria have adapted and have become immune to penicillin. Today, other antibiotics must be used. We are barely able to keep ahead of nature's ability to develop resistance to our antibiotics.

Chlamydia, although very prevalent, was not recognized as a diagnosable disease by culture or microscopy early on, since the organism was too small to be seen under the microscope. In the 1950s, it was difficult to culture. Chlamydia Trachomatis or just Trachoma was recognized as an eye disease by the cobblestone appearance of the conjunctiva and was treated by scraping the eyelids. When tetracycline became available, the treatment was much simplified.

Special cultures are now available and have become standard as part of a pelvic evaluation. The disease remains widespread and is probably the most commonly sexually transmitted sexual disease in our current time.

When I first started medical school, venereal warts were recognized as a slightly different kind of wart, located in the genital area. They were treated by a variety of destructive procedures using chemicals, cautery, and freezing. At that time, the correlation with cancer of the cervix had not been made.

We learned to do Pap smears as part of a gynecological exam in the 1950s. They were not as strongly recommended on a yearly basis as they are now. Georgios Papanicolaou first developed the test in the late 1940s. Slowly, physicians began to recognize the value of this test in recognizing early changes that would eventually lead to cancer of the cervix. There were several types of venereal warts that could be typed with DNA studies as the years went by. Only a few had the ability to cause the cancerous cervical changes. The warts were easily spread during sexual contact. Since they were caused by the human papilloma virus, the destructive procedures were not always curative. The warts would frequently return and spread around the rectum, labia, and penis requiring re-treatment.

We have made great strides in caring for the many facets of early detection of cervical cancer. After a few years in practice, I had to learn how to perform colposcopy so that the mildly abnormal Pap smears could be more fully evaluated. This involved using a binocular microscope that had a longer focal length. The physician could examine the cervix of a woman and see minor changes that were present but not visible to the naked eye without 60 power magnification. We could then direct our attention to those areas and take selected biopsies and scrapings for further evaluation.

Treatment could also be done with a freezing device to destroy the abnormal tissue. Recently, a vaccine has been developed, allowing young girls to be immunized against the HPV, or human papilloma virus. Perhaps we can eradicate the disease of cervical cancer in the future.

CHAPTER 15
THE DIPHTHERIA OUTBREAK

On December 21, l961, the Edwards family presented themselves to the hospital ER with complaints of sore throats, fever, and malaise. They lived out of town in the Sarpy hills, so they didn't see the doctor very often, unless it was something a little more serious. This proved to be the case.

There were three children, all complaining of sore throats and hoarseness. It was immediately obvious that Tom, the three year old, was the sickest. He was pale, lethargic, feverish, and had a fetid smell about him. When I examined his throat, there was a gray white exudate covering his tonsils and into the back part of his throat. His neck glands were also swollen and he was having some difficulty with his breathing.

Although I had never seen a case of diphtheria, I was sure that this was the real thing and not just a case of strep throat. I asked the parents if the children had been immunized against diphtheria, tetanus, and whooping cough with the DPT shots that most children get as they are growing up. The answer was "No."

I tried to peel off the membrane, but it was pretty adherent. I was able to get some of the purulent material and spread it on a slide to be examined under the microscope. I cultured the rest on Loeffler's media. Additional cultures were taken from the other two children and were sent to the state lab for confirmation.

The smear showed the small gram positive rods with small nodules on them characteristic of the diphtheria bacillus. We immediately put

Tom in a croup tent with oxygen, gave him a penicillin injection and 20,000 units of diphtheria antitoxin in each hip. Thank goodness that we had the antitoxin on hand, since that is the most important part of the treatment.

Diphtheria does not really invade the tissues like other bacteria, but grows locally on the surface and forms a spreading membrane that obstructs the airway. The toxin is formed in the membrane and diffuses into the body causing severe damage to the heart and other organs. Penicillin, although it kills the bacteria, doesn't really shorten the length of illness. The antitoxin and attention to protecting the airway is the key to preventing death.

It took only a short time to see that Tom was going to need a tracheotomy or he would suffocate. I had done a few tracheotomies while on the TB service in my residency, but that was with lots of staff around and an anesthetist to assist. We had none of these in our small hospital.

I called the parents aside and said, "Tom's trachea is closing off and if we don't get him into surgery and put a tube in his windpipe soon, he won't be able to breathe." "Red" Edwards, the father, said, "Can you do it here or will you have to take him to Billings?" "We don't have time to get him there, so I'll have to do it here," I replied. "Doctor, promise me that you won't let him die," Mrs. Edwards said. "I won't," I replied, "but we will have to act fast."

I took Tom into the surgery room and with the help of Mr. Halls and a nurse, we prepared Tom for surgery. I couldn't use any sedation since he was already having trouble breathing through his compromised airway. We mummified Tom by wrapping a sheet around him to restrain his arms and legs, and then cleaned off his neck. I injected local anesthesia, and then made a small vertical incision in the mid-line of his neck with the nurse holding his head steady. I then spread the subcutaneous tissue away from the trachea. There are a lot of blood vessels in this area, and any bleeding only makes the job more difficult. Time was of the essence.

The tracheotomies that I had done previously were all on adults where the structures were much larger. Here was this three year old, struggling for his next breath. Talk about pressure! Finally, the tracheal rings were exposed and Mr. Halls had the retractors in just the right place. I cut through two of the cartilaginous rings and slipped a small skin hook on one side so that I wouldn't lose the exposure. I cut a small piece of the tracheal cartilage away. There wasn't much room, but I was able to slide the metal tracheotomy tube into the trachea and remove the guide.

We were rewarded with a gush of air and relaxation of Tom's tense body. I placed a few sutures to partially close the skin, and then we attached the cotton cords to the side of the tube and tied them in the back of his neck so the tube would stay secure. Now it was up to the antitoxin and good nursing care.

He was placed back in the mist tent with oxygen and his vital signs were monitored. What I would have given for one of our modern day monitors that measures blood pressure, pulse, respirations, oxygen level, and EKG, all without disturbing the patient. But that was then, and this is now. Tom's color had now improved, and his pulse had dropped from 140 to 100. I called the parents into his room and said, "I think he'll be okay now." We all gave a sigh of relief.

I was feeling pretty good about him, but now I had to finish up the other two children. They were both given penicillin shots and antitoxin. Since they were breathing normally and were not as severe, they were sent home.

Shick tests were applied to everyone. This is a skin test that injects a small amount of toxin into the skin. If a person has immunity either from an immunization or naturally, no reaction occurs. If a person has no immunity, the area becomes very red at the end of two days. Mr. and Mrs. Edwards were both given penicillin and started on diphtheria-tetanus immunizations. The next day I got in touch with the Public Health Nurse about the diphtheria outbreak. She went to the school and began getting throat cultures on all the students in Tom's, and his siblings' classes. Then she gave DPT boosters to a number of the children.

Tom made steady improvement and the tracheotomy tube was removed four days later. He missed Christmas at home, but made it home for New Years. That was the best Christmas present that the family could have.

Diphtheria was first described as early as 400 B.C. by Hippocrates. It has taken the lives of countless numbers of people since that time, but was especially lethal in young children. There was really no treatment until a physician, Joseph O'Dwyer, developed the tracheotomy tube in the 1880s. Dr. Klebs first described the bacteria in 1883. In 1890, Emil Von Behring developed a horse serum antitoxin which dramatically helped counteract the effects of the toxin produced by the bacteria. Dr. Loeffler developed a horse serum culture medium, and this formula was still used when I cultured Tom Edwards.

Tracheotomies are rarely done in our current medical environment since it is easier to intubate someone and put them on a ventilator than to do a tracheotomy. When I started practice in Hardin there was no such thing as a ventilator, or at least not in a small hospital. I only encountered diphtheria once more in my career and that was in a school teacher. Her case was mild and did not require hospitalization, but only antitoxin and antibiotics.

I wonder today if doctors would recognize the grayish membrane in the throat as diphtheria. Our current generation of physicians probably has never had the dubious honor of encountering this disease in their practice of medicine.

Time marches on!

CHAPTER 16
THE CLINIC

It soon became apparent that Marlene and I would have to start looking for a house, since our daughter Lois, was a fussy baby and cried a lot at night. We worried that we would be disturbing the other residents at Koebbe's apartments. Besides, we needed to feel more settled down.

One incident that spurred us toward getting a house occurred one afternoon when we tied our Pug, Spike, to the water faucet serving the front lawn of the apartment house. We had acquired Spike in Salinas after Smiley passed on. Marlene's parents had flown to Salinas in Tony's plane to be with us and help out after Marlene's delivery. She went overdue, and when Marlene and Dora were walking on the streets of Salinas, there was a man with a pug puppy for sale for thirty dollars. Dora thought that would be good company for Marlene so they bought him. He was probably the best pug that we have had in the long line of pugs during our lifetime. Well, anyway, Spike was running back and forth on the long leash and in the process he turned the faucet on, letting the water run unattended for several hours. It flooded the lawn, which was fairly new, and the ground sunk down a few inches. We were quite embarrassed and now realized that Spike would need a back yard somewhere to run unfettered by a leash.

Houses were in short supply, since the large numbers of people who worked at the Yellowtail Dam project had swelled the population of Hardin, Fort Smith, and St. Xavier. Marlene's father was helpful in knowing what to look for in a house as far as basements, plumbing, and general construction of the available houses. Marlene, Tony, and Dora, his wife, began house hunting while I was busy from early morning to late at night with the practice.

They found a three bedroom house with an unfinished basement and we soon moved in. With that problem out of the way, the next step was to find a better place than the Kronmiller building for the extremely busy practice. We had been promised that if I moved to Hardin, a clinic would be built to house two doctors. This never happened, so I started looking for a contractor to build a new clinic. Mr. Wallin (Wally) was more than happy to arrange financing at the Big Horn County State Bank.

I was put in touch with a firm, Erdman and Associates, which specialized in building medical buildings. Soon we were breaking ground on two lots adjacent to the hospital. This was to be their first clinic in Montana, and they were very careful to have a successful relationship with me, and also to build a clinic that would show off their expertise.

Things went well without delays or problems during the construction. Within four months we were moved in and able to see many more patients in an efficient manner. The Clinic had six exam rooms, an x-ray room, a lab, a good sized waiting room, and a business office. I had also added another nurse, a secretary, a bookkeeper, and a cleaning lady to my staff.

The next item on the agenda was to get another doctor to join the practice. The forty patients a day, four operations a week, ten deliveries and thirty admissions a month, in addition to every night in the emergency room was getting to be pretty tiring. On my Thursday afternoons off, I would go to Billings to get supplies and discuss cases and x-rays with doctors there. I would arrive home to find an emergency room filled with patients who were waiting for me to return. Things had to change!

Fortunately, one of the doctors in my residency, Jim Miech, was finishing his two year military service obligation. He joined the practice, but I'll talk more about that when I cover the chapter on the doctors of Hardin later. Since the clinic was just adjacent to the hospital, it made things very efficient to run over for emergencies, or to check an obstetrical patient, without leaving the office patients waiting for long periods.

Things were looking up!

CHAPTER 17
THE DIXIELANDERS

After we had settled in to Hardin for a few months, we began to get acquainted with many of the people. Leroy (Wally) Wallin was president of the Big Horn County State Bank, and was instrumental in getting us to Hardin after our first meeting on our plane ride survey of Montana. We were invited over for dinner and soon discovered that we were both musicians and had a lot in common. Wally had even played a few times as a fill in musician with "Red Nichols and the Five Pennies" earlier in his career.

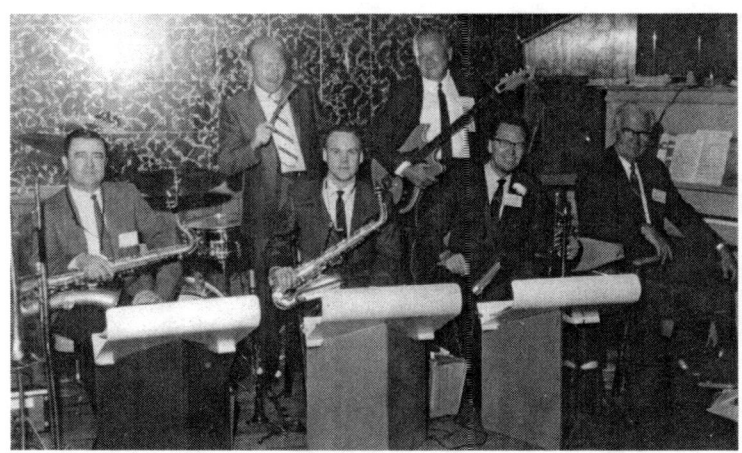

The Dixilanders

We thought it would be fun to organize a small band and play for benefits around town. He played trumpet, and I played alto sax and clarinet. We found that Doug Freeman, a lawyer in town played tenor sax and trombone, and Joe Nurre, an insurance man played drums, and later learned bass. We shopped around for a piano player and finally got Ken Fox, of Fox Oil, to be our fifth member. I had a considerable amount of music that I saved from the small dance band that I had in college, so we started practicing. For the smooth dance numbers, we used two saxophones and trumpet to get three part harmony. For the dixieland tunes, we used trumpet, clarinet, and trombone, along with drums and piano. Over the course of the next twenty years we probably raised over $30,000 for various charities and benefits.

Over the years, illness and death caused me to replace most of the members. Wally, and then Ken Fox, died of heart attacks and were replaced by Ken Boggio, the high school band director on trumpet, and Karen Enzminger, an excellent pianist, who was a nurse at the clinic. Joe Nurre died from pancreatic cancer and was replaced by Vince Hurtig on electric bass. Finally, Doug passed on from complications of multiple small strokes, and was replaced by Linda Troyer on clarinet. Being in the band didn't seem to bode well for the health of its members!

We had a tradition of opening the deer season with a dance at Sayle, Montana. It was a small ranching community in the heart of nowhere about sixty miles east of Hardin. They would have a box lunch social where the women made a box lunch, the men would bid on them and then have the first dance. This raised money for some of their community activities.

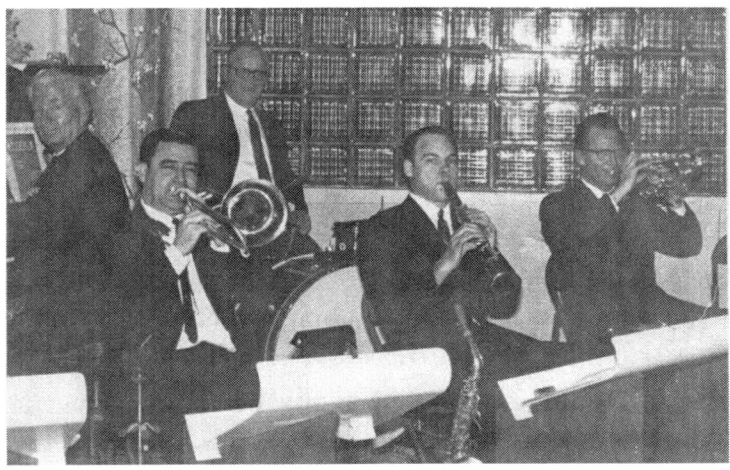

The Dixilanders. Ken, Doug, Joe, Me, Wally

96

We stayed at "the BARN" which was owned by Ken's brother, Chick. It could sleep about a dozen people in rather simple style. The following morning after the dance we would rise for an early breakfast of eggs, bacon, and hash browns, cooked by Bud Harris, and then go out for the deer hunt. I remember one of the first hunts that I was part of at Sayle. I owned a 30.06 with a four power scope, and as we were surveying the landscape at sun up, I saw the profile of a deer about 150 yards away just clearing the breast of the hill. I took aim and fired and the deer disappeared. A few seconds later it reappeared in the same place and I wondered if I had fired high. I took aim again and fired, and the deer disappeared again. We walked up the hill and just as we cleared the summit I saw, to my surprise, two dead deer very close together. It was lucky that I had both an "A" and "B" tag that day.

As long as I am on the subject of the outdoors and hunting, I might as well include a few more hunting stories here. I had started archery hunting in Minnesota but never made a kill there. We had a group of archers in Hardin and we would camp in the Little Belt Mountains each year to hunt elk.

On one occasion I decided not to make the long ascent to the top of one of our favorite places where there was usually a lot of elk sign showing activity. Instead, I planned to strike out on my own to hunt some of the lower clear cuts and "parks" or open spaces on the mountain side. Since I was seeing nothing in the form of tracks or elk droppings, I decided to rest and catch my breath at the edge of one of the clear cuts.

Suddenly, I heard branches breaking and hoof beats. My heart was in my throat. I nocked an arrow just as about a dozen elk broke into the clearing at the other side about forty yards away. There were no bulls in the group, but I was after meat and not antlers. I selected a cow elk that was broadside about forty yards away, drew back my bowstring and aimed for the chest.

Just as I released the arrow she took a step forward, and by the time the arrow arrived, she was two feet further ahead. The arrow struck her just in front of the back leg. She took off running into the timber in a downhill direction. It didn't look like a kill shot, and one of the rules in archery is that one must always track a wounded animal to try to get another shot if it lies down later.

I got to the spot of the contact and soon spotted a blood trail. There was a significant amount of blood every five or six feet and I kept to the trail of broken branches and blood as it wound its way down the hill. At the bottom of the mountain, just on the edge of the meadow, I saw her lying down. There was no movement so I nocked another arrow and slowly approached her. I found that she was dead and that the arrow had hit her in the femoral artery, just in front of her left leg and she had bled out after running all the way downhill to a spot where I could drive my Bronco. I could load her up without the exhausting task of dragging her a quarter of a mile downhill. That was an easy hunt!

There were some good deer hunts also. I remember one in particular. I had a friend, Max Blanchard, who had taken up archery but had never made a hunt before. I told him we would go hunting on the property owned by John Walborn, a rancher who lived just west of Lame Deer, Montana. There were "coulees" where we could walk on each side and see if any deer were bedded down. They would usually break out on the opposite side if they were disturbed. I selected a likely ravine and we started out, one on each side. We hadn't walked more than a quarter of a mile when the biggest buck with the most magnificent set of antlers that I have ever seen spotted me. He stood up to make a run for it, but did not see Max, who was only twenty yards away on the opposite side, since all the deer's attention was entirely focused on me.

Max drew back and let his arrow fly, striking the buck in the chest just back of the front leg. The buck just dropped down again in his tracks and I let fly another arrow striking him in the other side of the chest. A few more death throes and he lay still. When we dressed him out, we found that Max's arrow had pierced his heart for a perfect kill shot. The deer weighed just about 300 pounds. Max said, "This bow hunting is great fun, and really pretty easy."

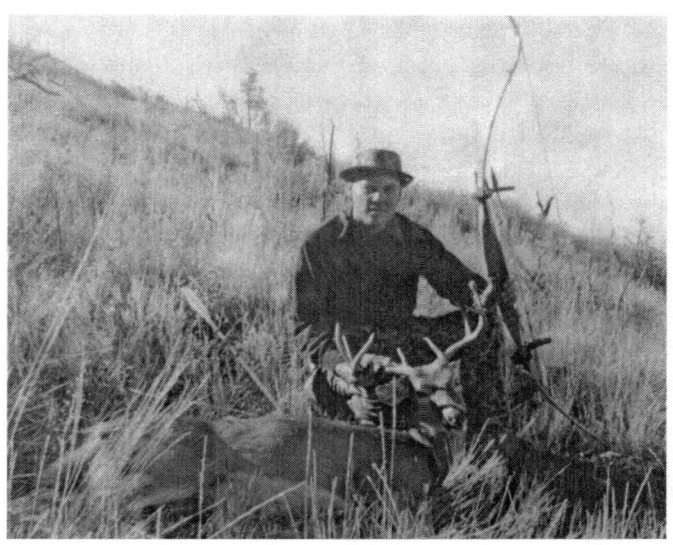

Deer Hunting in the Missouri Breaks

I remember another elk hunt, my first with a rifle. At that time my rifle was a 30-30 which is a little under-powered for elk. I also carried my .45 revolver on my hip for my "just in case gun." I was hunting with Pastor Paul Lee from our church and two other friends, but we had separated to cover more ground in the Missouri breaks. I was walking along an old logging road, moving slowly and carefully to avoid any unnecessary noise, when I heard a twig snap. I dropped down to a crouch and spotted a young two point bull coming up from lower ground.

He was in a grove of small aspen trees. I couldn't get a clear shot, since he was almost directly facing me and there were too many trees. The distance was about thirty five yards and I had open sights on my rifle. I finally decided that I would aim directly at a three inch sapling that was lined up with the front profile of the elk's head. I pulled the trigger and the elk jerked back and began shaking his head back and forth, and then he went down. After being dazed for a second, he started to get up. I ran up to the elk as I was pulling out my revolver. I got there before he could fully regain his senses. Just as he regained his feet, I fired again with two head shots and it was all over. I went back to reassess the "crime scene" and found that my bullet had pierced the

99

sapling exactly in the center and then hit the elk in the nose, stunning it temporarily. That gave me just enough time to get close enough for my .45 to finish the job. That turned out to be the only elk encounter of the weekend for our group.

As long as I am on hunting stories, I might as well relate a rather unusual water fowl hunt. I was on a small island in the Big Horn river, hunting ducks as they would fly by over some shallow water into which I could wade to retrieve any fallen birds. There were a fair number of Mallards that would fly by giving me some good opportunities to get my limit, and I was having a great time.

There was a single goose that kept flying in circles very high up above the island. In retrospect, I suspect that its mate had been shot by someone earlier and that it was searching. Geese mate for life, unlike ducks. The goose was probably fifty yards straight up above me, and essentially out of range for a shotgun, even a long barrel 12 gauge with magnum 3 inch shells and #2 shot. The goose was giving a rather plaintive call and I decided to take a shot even though I knew I had little chance of reaching it at that range.

I brought my shotgun to my shoulder, gave the goose a little "Kentucky windage" and pulled the trigger. The goose ceased its forward flight and with wings askew, came screaming to earth cartwheeling like a Zero shot down by antiaircraft fire. It hit with a thud about 20 feet in front of me. When I had recovered it, I began to search for the wound that brought it down, but there was no blood or pellet that I could see for the fatal wound. I had pulled out a number of feathers to see if a pellet had pierced the heart, but again, nothing. Finally, I looked carefully at the head and notice an entry wound of a single pellet just below the eye that had gone into the brain and brought down the goose.

It was probably fitting that it didn't have to suffer the loss of its mate very long. And now, it's time to get back to medicine.

CHAPTER 18
THE "DRUGGIES"

Mind altering substances have been used for as long as mankind has come down from the trees and walked upright. Alcohol was probably the first to be used in a meaningful way, but certain hallucinogenic mushrooms, coca leaves, marijuana, and the poppy plant became a part of the culture far back into antiquity. These drugs were used both as recreational, and also in medical treatments in early medicine.

Before we had anesthetics, whiskey and laudanum (tincture of opium) were the major sources of pain relief in surgical operations and injuries. Opium was smoked in the Far East, and found its way into many of the early pharmaceuticals of early medicine. Lydia Pinkham's tonic contained a high percentage of alcohol. A few years back, I was told that opium was also included. I could not substantiate the latter ingredient, even with an extensive review, but it would make sense that it did contain opium since both pain and cramps could be relieved. It was touted as a relief for almost any "female" complaint. Addiction to opiates as a result of unknown inclusions in some of these herbal remedies was undoubtedly present, but not recognized or discussed in polite society.

A review of these drugs and how they have gone from legitimate to illegitimate is probably in order. Alcohol had always been accepted as part of humanity's culture, especially in the United States. In 1919, the Volstad Act and the Eighteenth Amendment were enacted making it a crime to possess alcohol even for the purpose of drinking it in the home. The history of prohibition is well known to all of you, so I will not go into it further at this time.

Coca has been used by natives of South America since antiquity. The natives would chew the leaves to give themselves more energy and produce an elevation of mood.

When the Spanish conquistadors were forcing the native slaves to work in the gold fields, they found it necessary to supply the natives with coca leaves in order to get them to work in a productive manner.

In the 1500s coca was brought back to Europe and introduced to the general population. Eight percent of the Europeans living in Peru were involved in the coca trade.

In the 1800s, the first poem about coca was written by Abraham Cowley titled "A Legend of Coca." It was found that there were medicinal uses for coca, and in 1855, cocaine hydrochloride was first extracted from the leaves. It was used as a topical anesthetic for the eye and also in the nose and throat. It could be used in the nose to shrink swollen tissues and constrict blood vessels in the case of nosebleeds.

In 1886, John Pemberton introduced Coca Cola, which contained about 60 mg. of cocaine per serving. It was not removed from the popular drink until about 1903. The severity of cocaine addiction was not really recognized since it could be purchased over the counter. In 1912, the US Government reported 5,000 deaths from cocaine use. That was with a population only one-third of what it is today. The Pure Food and Drug Act of 1906 required listing all ingredients on patent medicines since statistics showed that somewhere between one-fourth to one-half million people were addicted to narcotics by the turn of the century. This act led to the demise of the patent medicine industry.

German chemists, in an effort to find a less addicting drug than morphine for addicts trying to break the habit, synthesized Heroin. This turned out to be a disaster since it was even more addicting. The Harrison Act, enacted in 1914, imposed a stamp of illegitimacy on narcotic use, and the Supreme Court held that doctors could not prescribe narcotics to taper addicts. Prevention of withdrawal symptoms was deemed not a legitimate medical procedure, and doctors could be prosecuted if they instituted treatment. Clinics to treat addiction were shut down which led the addicts to the underworld for their drugs.

Snorting cocaine became popular in about 1905. Nasal damage occurred and was described in the medical literature in 1910. Freebase cocaine was first developed in the 1970s and was popularized by dealers and glamorized by Hollywood. It was discovered that cocaine hydrochloride could be converted to a smokable form by heating it in a solution of baking soda, thus making a freebase which volatilized easily when heated and then could be smoked. When it is being heated, it makes a crackling sound, thus the name "crack cocaine."

Marijuana was used in China 5,000 years ago as an anesthetic. It was also used to control muscle spasms, pain, and indigestion. In the 1800s, the American medical profession used it for spastic conditions, headaches, labor pains, and menstrual cramps.

Since the more recent history of marijuana is fairly well-known, I won't go into it except to relate a somewhat interesting anecdote that happened to me. Our family has a cabin on the Stillwater River near Nye, Montana. As my son-in-law and I were walking along the river bank just below a vacant house, we noticed three healthy plants about three to four feet tall that looked just like pictures that I had seen of marijuana. We pulled them up and brought them home to evaluate further.

I called the Sheriff's office to let him know that we would be bringing them in for identification before transporting them in the car. I could just see getting into an accident with three big marijuana plants in the back seat and trying to explain to the Highway Patrolman that I was bringing them in for identification. I am sure he would have said, "I've heard that story before. Surely you can make up a better one than that." In any event, I got them to the Sheriff and he did identify them and took custody of them.

That brings me to all of the excuses that I have heard over the years about why my patients needed refills on their narcotics before it was time to have used up their supply. Some of these are listed below.

    1. They fell in the toilet.
    2. They fell in the sink.
    3. My purse was stolen.

4. My husband, sister, brother, stole them.
5. My husband threw them away.
6. The pharmacist didn't give me the full amount.
7. They fell out of the car and the tire ran over them.
8. The dog chewed up the container.
9. I had to double up since the pain was too severe.
10. The car was broken into and my pills were stolen.

Patients from other areas frequently come into the emergency room with complaints of pain that are hard to challenge such as migraine headaches and back pain. They usually gave an allergy history to all the drugs that we might use except the one that they were after to sell on the street. Sometimes they were fortunate enough with their hard luck story to wheedle out a dozen or so pills of oxycodone.

Frequently, the story will be that they are traveling on the weekend and their doctor in another state or town is not available to verify the medical history. The pain is usually of a type that cannot be verified with physical diagnosis. A compassionate doctor does not want a patient to be refused pain relief for a legitimate complaint, but we don't want to be taken advantage of either. We now have inter-hospital communication between hospitals in the same general area when we suspect a patient of fraud, and memos are sent alerting Emergency Departments of these situations.

I remember several cases where drug seekers were traveling down the highway and stopping at every small town between Bozeman, Montana, and Denver, Colorado, with the same story. They could acquire quite a stash of pills, usually obtained on credit from the hospital. They could then sell them for five to ten dollars a pill. When confronted, they were usually gone before the police could become involved.

We have to be very careful with our prescription pads in today's environment and we cannot leave pads lying around the ER as we did a decade or two ago. We use duplicate prescriptions now so that they cannot alter the number of pills on the prescription. I have had pharmacists call me asking if I really wanted two hundred oxycodones for a patient when my duplicate copy showed twenty.

The last story that I want to relate in this chapter occurred a number of years ago when amphetamines were becoming the most popular trendy drug. We didn't really appreciate the potential for addiction, and the pharmaceutical salesmen were encouraging us to prescribe the latest diet pill, Dexadrine. Ten or fifteen milligrams of this in a timed release form was guaranteed not only to kill one's appetite for twelve hours, but it also gave the tired housewife energy to get her house cleaned and all the other chores that she just couldn't get to. Truck drivers also found that they could drive for longer periods without getting sleepy, which seemed to be a better alternative than lots of coffee.

Dexedrine caused some people to be a little jittery, and for those people there was Dexamyl, which contained a little barbiturate in it to take the edge off. We jokingly said the pill had one ingredient to speed them up and another to slow them down, so the net result was neutrality. Dexedrine was a regularly prescribed prescription by most of us in the '60s. In all honesty, dextroamphetamine did not carry the same potential for addiction as methamphenamine, and no one thought about the potential of injecting it for a greater rush.

Well, back to the story. A deputy sheriff brought in a twenty or so year old male who was high on dextroamphetamine and was jumping in front of cars and trucks on the highway causing a significant traffic hazard. They sat him down in the emergency room and then left for another part of the hospital. I began to interview the patient when he suddenly got up and said, "I'm leaving."

One thing that I remember being told about people high on drugs was, "Don't block the door." Well, there was no one else around except me, so I immediately blocked the door and said, "No you're not." He either took a swing at me or tried to push me aside, so I caught his wrist, spun him around, and put a full Nelson wrestling hold on him and slammed him down on the gurney. I then called out in a rather loud voice, "I need a little help in here."

The deputies arrived and handcuffed him in preparation to taking him up to the psychiatric ward in Billings. He was pretty wild by that time, so I had to sedate him with some IV Valium. When a person is high on drugs, he doesn't like needles, so my patient was screaming, "I'm gonna kill you all and especially you, Dr. Whiting." I figured that by the time he had been detoxed and probably sent to Warm Springs for treatment, he would have forgotten all about the episode.

The next morning I called the psychiatrist to see how he was doing for what I was expecting to be an extended stay. I was a little surprised when the psychiatrist said, "Oh, I dismissed him this morning." Needless to say, I looked over my shoulder more than once in the ensuing several weeks.

CHAPTER 19
THE PREEMIES

Neonatal care is now a specialty, but in the 1960s there were no neonatal intensive care nurseries. At that time we really didn't have the technology and tools for the invasive monitoring and evaluation of these tiny babies that is present today. We couldn't monitor heart rate, EKG, respiration, oxygen level, blood pressure, and temperature on a few fancy machines with flashing lights and beeping noises as we do today. There were no tiny flexible intravenous catheters and microdrips for fluid administration as we have today. We really didn't understand respiratory distress syndrome of the newborn, nor how best to treat it. Babies either made it or they didn't, depending on how mature their lungs were.

The first breath that a newborn takes is a huge effort. The air sacs are closed at birth and with that first mighty effort and first breath, they open up and stay inflated. Subsequent breaths don't require the same effort and expenditure of energy. With respiratory distress the lungs sacs don't stay open, and with exhalation, they close up again, requiring more effort and energy to keep breathing. Eventually, the baby tires, and finally stops breathing. Today, these preemies would be intubated and put on a respirator to assist their breathing, and would be given surfactant, which keeps their air sacs open. But this was the world of the 1960s.

My patient Mildred W. presented to the hospital on February 6, 1962, in premature labor with ruptured membranes and labor contractions. She was only six months along. She was already dilated enough so that stopping her labor was not possible. Delivery was imminent and we would be expecting a very tiny premature infant that would probably not survive. Whether or not the baby's lungs were mature enough would be the deciding factor. Transferring the mother 48 miles to Billings at this stage of labor would entail too much risk, and there was no special premature nursery there anyway.

Labor went rapidly and we were soon in the delivery room where a tiny female made her entrance into the world. She was wiped off, and with the stimulation of this procedure, she took her first breath and let out a weak cry to announce her presence. We immediately placed her in the incubator to keep her warm, and started some low flow oxygen. She weighed one pound and twelve ounces. She looked so frail and fragile. "Will she make it," Mildred said in a halting voice. "Please save her." "She is tiny but she seems strong," I replied. Now we had to watch and see if she would continue to breathe easily or would begin to struggle as the hours passed. The treatment was simply to keep her warm, with just enough oxygen to satisfy her needs. Too much oxygen could cause damage to the eyes with proliferation of blood vessels in the retina.

After a few hours we tried to feed her a small amount of glucose water by gavage tube, so that she did not need to expend any energy by sucking or swallowing. She tolerated it okay, so the next step was to try some dilute Nutramagen, a special predigested formula. We had to aspirate her stomach each time we fed her to ascertain if there was any residual formula still present, and then we could plan how much to increase the feeding. Things seemed to go okay although she lost a little more weight as expected over the next several days. Finally, she leveled off and began to gain. It looked like she was over the hump and would make it. But then catastrophe struck.

It was about noon, and I was going to get a bite in the hospital dining room to save a little time for the afternoon rush of patients. I walked past the nursery and as I looked through the glass, I saw that Cynthia, (she had been named by then) was not her nice pink color, but instead, was purple. I rushed into the nursery and quickly snatched Cynthia out of the incubator and placed her on the flat work table. She was not breathing and her stomach was markedly distended.

Her heart rate was about 40, but I didn't bother listening for more than a second or two. I took a feeding tube and quickly slipped it into her stomach and aspirated about 15 cc. of air and a little milk. This took the pressure away from her diaphragm and allowed her lungs to more easily expand. We did not have a mask small enough to ventilate her so I quickly placed my mouth over her nose and mouth and gave a little puff of air. I then gently squeezed her tiny chest with two fingers. It is hard to calculate how much or how hard to blow into a preemie of this size to inflate the lungs. Too much pressure and the lungs could be ruptured, and too little, no air gets in at all. Another puff and then I observed for a few seconds. Heart rate 50, but still no breathing.

"Come on, little one. You came into this world way too soon, but it's not time for you to leave," I said to myself. Then, finally, I heard a small gasp, and then another. Heart rate 54. Then a breath, and then a cry. Heart rate 70. A feeling of both joy and relief came over me as the color and muscle tone seemed to flow back into the baby. Now I could stop holding my breath as she started to breathe regularly. It was lucky that I happened to be walking by, because the nurse that usually monitored the nursery from the nurse's station had been called to a patient's room, and for those few minutes, no one was watching. We had dodged a bullet, but now I wondered if she would be brain damaged and end up with a disability.

We observed her carefully for the next few hours and then gave her another small gavage feeding which she tolerated well. She gave us no further problems. We discharged her when she weighed about five pounds. I was rewarded seventeen years later with a beautiful senior prom picture of her in a white formal gown.

On May 20, 1962, my patient Evelyn F. who was pregnant with twins arrived at the hospital in active labor, at not quite seven months along in her pregnancy. This was a replay of the case from a few months before, so the nurses were ready for what we might experience. Again, we could not stop her labor, so we readied ourselves for the expected tiny babies.

Twin deliveries are a little more complicated than single births, and premature babies added an additional risk. The first baby presented head first, and this was a blessing, since the head is the largest part of the baby to go through the birth canal, making it easier for the shoulders and body to follow. The baby was suctioned and cried soon after, saying, "Here I am." A few minutes later the second baby crowned, with a head first presentation and delivered, followed by a lusty cry. I felt that these babies would have a good chance to survive, despite their small size. They weighed 2 pounds, 7 1/4 ounces, and 2 pounds, 6 1/2 ounces. We instituted the same measures with low flow oxygen, gavage feedings, and careful monitoring, and slowly they began to gain weight. At about 5 pounds, James and Jocquiline were discharged from the hospital. I received a graduation picture of these two attractive young adults just after their eighteenth birthdays.

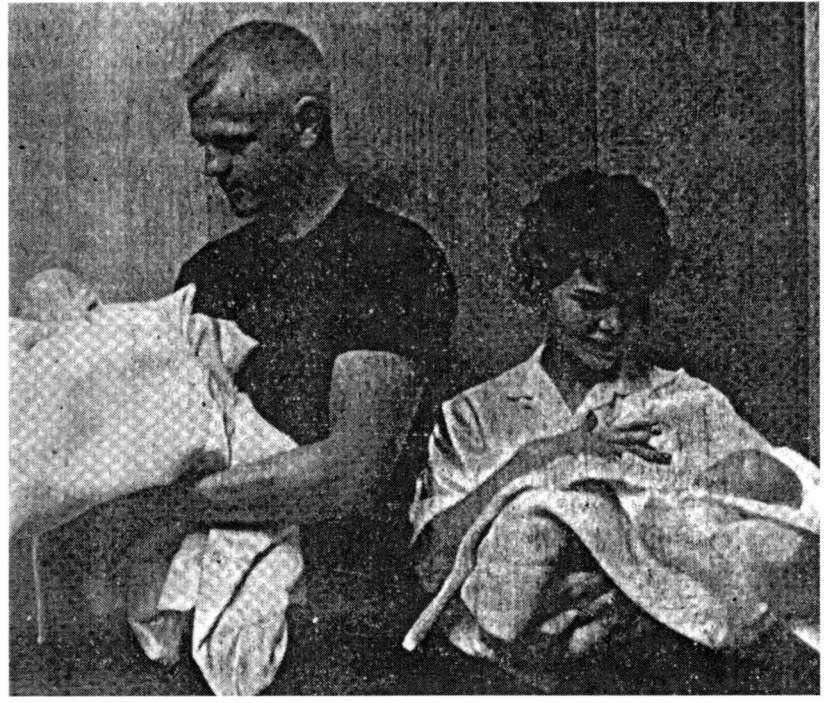

The twins

We had other premature births during my obstetrical career, but these were the smallest. When Billings established a premature nursery, we transferred our premature babies to that hospital by helicopter, after stabilization, umbilical catheter insertion, and IV fluids, following the protocol that had been established in later years.

CHAPTER 20
HYPNOSIS

There is a lot to know about hypnosis besides stage entertainment and parlor tricks, and much of this relates to medicine. Before I tell you about all the medical uses that I have both seen and done, I need to explain some of the history relating to its discovery and use.

Hypnotism has been present in one form or another since very early times. It was used in the sleep temples of ancient Egypt and was even spoken about by Hippocrates. Various ways to induce the state included chanting, drumming, incantations, and hand passing. Various ways of inducing a hypnotic trance were done by Druids, Vikings, Hindu priests, and holy men of many religions in past ages.

Modern hypnosis probably first began in 1773, with the efforts of Franz Anton Mesmer, a German physician, who was treating a patient complaining of a variety of recurrent physical and psychosomatic ailments. He was operating under the assumption that planets, tides, and a magnetic fluid that coursed through the universe were the basis of human disease. By redirecting the magnetic flow, he felt that he could alter the disequilibrium and then cure the patient. He called this animal magnetism and he attracted a large following of patients which antagonized the medical community.

The French Royal Commission of 1774 discredited him and explained his apparent cures were due to patients with overly active imaginations. Coupled with this and several well dramatized failures, he rapidly fell from grace and lived out the remainder of his life in obscurity. Although he disappeared from view, his ideas did not.

The idea of a fluid magnetic force was discarded and the subsequent physicians came to realize that the success of the procedure was related to the belief of the patients in their therapist. James Braid, a Scottish neurosurgeon, became interested in the procedure after observing demonstrations by a traveling mesmerizer and he began lecturing on it in 1841.

He coined the term hypnotism, considering it a form of nervous sleep. He used the method of fixing on a bright object about 18 inches in front of the eyes to induce the trance. As time passed, there were reputable physicians who rescued hypnosis from a pseudoscience to a more reputable form of treatment, and found that there were a number of niches where hypnosis seemed to work. These included psychotherapy, anesthesia, and treating a variety of medical problems.

This leads me to my use of hypnosis which began in 1962. I had read a book by Dave Elman, a rather well recognized hypnotist, who showed that there were a number of medical conditions that could easily be benefited by hypnotic suggestions. He had laid out a course of about 18 hours of lectures on LP records which I purchased and began to study. These included using hypnosis for obstetrical deliveries, pain relief, smoking secession, local anesthesia for wound repair, stuttering, treatment of headaches, weight loss therapy, and relaxation therapy. Hypnosis could be used to benefit any number of these conditions.

Dorine, my nurse, had her first baby under general anesthesia and didn't wake up for some time after the delivery, causing her to miss everything that went on during the event. She wanted to have her second child under hypnosis, and wanted to have it free from pain. She said, "You'd better get good at this quickly so I can have a more pleasant experience than with my first child."

The procedure was to induce a trance with visualizing oneself as floating on a cloud and freeing all other thoughts from the mind. I would then suggest a deepening of this very relaxed feeling as the person drifted deeper into the hypnotic state. Loss of the ability to open one's eyes or move one's muscles, followed by anesthesia to pain was then suggested. This could be confirmed by pinching the skin with a surgical clamp or using a towel clip to actually pierce the skin, then asking the person to try to open her eyes or move her arm which, if the state was deep enough, would not occur. With practice, the state could be obtained more quickly with each session. For hypnosis to work, a willing subject is needed, who also recognizes the therapist as an authoritative figure. Physicians are good at being this kind of person.

Using hypnosis was an excellent way to have a relaxed, pain free delivery. It does take practice, just as the current La Maz method does, but it is much more effective. Dorine, two of the hospital nurses and my office manager, Glennine, all had their babies under hypnosis with excellent results. Once they are under, there is very little movement and the eyes remain closed throughout the entire labor. The patient is permitted to lighten up and move in order to use the bed pan or have a drink of water. Then she is put back in a deeper state again. We did not do very many exams to determine the dilatation of the cervix, since this required lightening up the hypnotic state. When Dorine was ready to deliver, the nurse said, "I saw her toe twitch so I thought she must be pretty far along," and sure enough, Dorine was completely dilated and ready to move to the delivery room. No local anesthesia was required for the episiotomy or the repair since the anesthesia of the area was suggested by hypnosis.

Myrna Eckleman, one of our hospital nurses, also had a delivery under hypnosis with similar results. She remarked that the experience was very pleasant, and although she was aware of everything in the labor room, there was no anxiety or discomfort. The attending nurses were always a little skittish about the procedure, since they could only see this peaceful, relaxed patient, with closed eyes and a slight smile on her face, while being about ready to deliver in the labor room bed.

The other patient that I remember who was an excellent subject was Mrs. Thompson, the director of nurses. She had a similar experience and we almost didn't get her into the delivery room in time. There were numerous others of my regular patients who also had similar good results, but you get the idea.

Many patients wanted hypnosis to help them stop smoking. The same technique was used to get them into a deeply suggestible state. I then gave them the suggestion that the cigarette would taste so bad that they would be unable to smoke it. Positive health suggestions were also given and the patients were told that no desire for a cigarette would occur. I then woke them up from the trance and asked them to light up a cigarette. One or two puffs and they would make a face and would extinguish the cigarette. I remember one cowboy who said, "Whooy, this tastes just like what I've been cleaning out of the horse stalls." The short term effects were quite good, but unless frequent follow up visits and reinforcements of the suggestions were given, relapse was likely to occur several weeks down the road. Probably, these patients were not really motivated, and wanted someone else to make them stop with no effort from themselves. Similar procedures were also used in weight loss efforts to curb the appetite and reduce hunger pangs.

I had a patient come into the emergency room one evening with the complaint that his right arm was paralyzed. Surely enough, the arm was completely limp, but had normal reflexes. I asked him to describe what happened. He related to me that he had gotten into an argument with his girl friend and became so angry that he raised his arm to strike her and the arm suddenly became paralyzed. It was immediately obvious to me that this was a case of hysterical paralysis. I put him in a trance and told him that when he awoke, full function of his arm would be present. When I snapped my fingers and told him to open his eyes, he was amazed that he could now use his arm. I explained to him the effect of the mind on our bodies, and then we had a little conference on anger management.

There was a patient in the nursing home who was dying of metastatic cancer and was in considerable pain from it. Increasing doses of narcotics were needed to control her symptoms. I decided to try to relieve her terminal cancer pain with hypnosis. She proved to be a good subject. Under hypnosis I gave her the suggestion that she would feel no further pain from the cancer and would need no further narcotics. Each time she felt any discomfort, she was to do the self induced trance and block the pain. Even though I had seen so many good results with hypnosis in such a variety of conditions, I was still amazed when she needed no further narcotics until she died from her cancer.

Hypnosis was a good tool in sewing up lacerations in children. I would use the technique of having them close their eyes and pretend that they could not open them, as I put them into a light trance. I gave them the suggestion that as long as their eyes remained closed, they could feel nothing that bothered them. It was important not to use any words such as stick, stitch, cut, pain, hurt, needle, or blood, so that no adverse pictures would form in their minds. I would then gently put in the anesthetic while I was continuing to remind that they could not open their eyes. I would then sew up the laceration with no crying or fear from the children. It was remarkable how relaxed and calm so many of these children would be.

There were also a few instances where I used hypnosis in the legal realm. Lupe Hernandez, Herman Rodriguez, and Benjamin Hernandez, Lupe's son, were driving on highway 47 north of Hardin on November 21, 1962, when they ran into the 27th car of a beet train where the tracks crossed the highway.

It was dark, and the windows were probably rolled up, so that they did not hear any noise from the rail cars when they collided with the train. Benjamin was thrown out and under the train and was killed instantly. Lupe was severely injured with a fractured pelvis, a concussion, and loss of consciousness for almost a week after the accident. When she awoke, she had total amnesia of the incident, and since the funeral was a closed casket service, she had no closure of the event.

Bob Wilson, the lawyer representing her, wanted to know what she remembered of the accident. She was a total blank, so he asked me if I would hypnotize her and try to restore her memory of the event. She agreed, I put her in a trance, and then regressed her back to the day of the accident. I then had her visualize the car driving down the highway and the events that followed. I felt that despite the concussion and loss of memory that could occur from trauma, we still might be able to unlock her memory of the event.

When we got to the part of hitting the train, she was screaming and crying as she relived the accident. I then gave her the suggestion that she would remember the event when she woke up from the trance. On awakening, she now had a clear memory of the accident which gave her closure of the event, and also information for Bob Wilson to use in his case against the railroad for a poorly marked crossing.

The last case that I want to discuss involves the use of hypnosis in law enforcement. Bob Wilson, County Attorney at the time, was investigating a fatality from a car accident involving three Crow Indians and one Cheyenne Indian, all of whom had been drinking heavily. They were driving at a high rate of speed when they went over one of the secondary train crossings and the car became airborne and crashed. One of the Crows was killed and the investigating officers needed to find out who was driving. The two surviving Crows immediately accused the Cheyenne of being the driver, and he could not remember anything of the accident with any clarity.

Joe Koebbe, one of the deputies, was instructed by Bob Wilson to bring the Cheyenne Indian to the clinic for hypnosis to see if we could reconstruct the events. I had really forgotten about this incident in later years, but Joe, who was present during the session, remembered clearly what happened, and he filled me in. The suspect was a good subject and easily went into a deep hypnotic state. Several tests were done to indicate that he was not faking anything before he was asked to live through the event again. He was able to go through the experience as if it was happening at the time, and he named one of the Crows as the driver. It must have been believable enough to the authorities, since he was released from any later prosecution.

Although hypnosis was a valuable tool in helping people with a variety of problems, as my practice became busier and busier, I began to phase it out due to time constraints that were required. It is used more by mental health professionals and psychiatric social workers now, but could be of value to anyone willing to put in the time to study the techniques, and benefits of the procedure.

CHAPTER 21
CANCER

During the past fifty years we have made great strides in our quest to conquer cancer. Now, we can frequently cure childhood leukemia, and with the advent of total body radiation followed by bone marrow transplant, adult leukemia also will frequently fall within our scope of cure.

We know how to attack cancer cells by starving them, cutting off their blood supply, or using multiple drug combinations to slow their growth. Radiation treatment can be focused to avoid healthy tissue and can destroy cancerous areas with great precision. Radioactive "seeds" or implants can be inserted into cancerous growths to shrink the size of tumors, which makes them more accessible to surgical removal.

Except for surgery and heavy doses of radiation, not much else was available when I started practice except for a few chemotheraputic agents. Radical surgery was the procedure of choice for breast cancer which included, in addition to removing the breast, removing the pectoralis major and pectoralis minor muscles and carrying the dissection into the axilla and stripping all of the lymphatics away so that the patient was frequently left with a chronically swollen arm requiring an elastic sleeve to reduce the persistent swelling. This was usually followed by super-voltage radiation which frequently caused skin burns and chronically damaged skin.

My mother had this procedure. Although she was cured of the breast cancer, she died thirty years later of lung cancer which I ascribed to the radiation to her chest wall. She was never a smoker, and she had no associated risk factors.

There were several remarkable cancer stories that I would like to talk about that defy what we would normally expect in those early years of my practice. Although I am sure that there were many to choose from, these four have always stuck in my mind.

Betty Jane, or B.J. as she was usually called, presented to me in September, 1963, with a distended abdomen that I immediately recognized as ascites, or free fluid in the peritoneal cavity. This is usually due to cirrhosis of the liver, but I knew that she was not a drinker. An X-ray showed the fine ground-glass appearance of fluid but not much else. We did not have the luxury of ultra sound, CT scan, or MRI at that time.

I inserted a large bore needle called a trochar into her abdomen and drained off about two quarts of yellow fluid and sent it for analysis. The report showed nonspecific abnormal cells. I scheduled her for surgery and when I opened her abdomen, I found a nightmare. She had a large cystadenocarcinoma of the left ovary with many tiny metastatic lesions spread throughout the pelvis, and also on the surface of the large and small bowel. I was able to remove the tumor, including the uterus, tubes and ovaries but was then left with what to do about the numerous metastatic lesions. I decided to use the cautery and to meticulously burn each lesion, one at a time. I destroyed about a hundred of the lesions before I was finished, but I worried that so much cautery on the surface of the bowel and on the peritoneal surfaces would leave her pretty sick for some time to come. Surprisingly, she healed up quickly and the ascites did not recur. Ovarian cancer which was this far advanced was usually a rapid death sentence, since it was impossible to get to all of the metastases.

At that time we did not have the chemotherapeudic agent Taxol to treat ovarian cancer, and this cancer is generally resistant to radiation.

BJ did not begin to show symptoms of ascites again until two years later. On January 27, 1965, I operated on her again and found the pelvis again riddled with metastatic lesions. There was a large cancerous growth attached to the surface of her bladder also. I made an elliptical incision around the tumor on the bladder, removed it, and then closed the bladder in three layers and inserted a catheter until it would have a chance to heal without distending or putting pressure on the suture lines. I started burning lesions again that were spread throughout the pelvis. I figured that if burning all those lesions had worked for two years, maybe I could buy her a little more time again.

B.J. stayed in the hospital for two weeks and kept the catheter for another ten days as an outpatient. She healed beautifully and remained symptom free with a productive life for six more years. In October, 1971, she entered the hospital for terminal care. She died October 22, 1971, more than eight years after she was initially found with far advanced disease.

Wilma Metcalf came to see me in August 1989 at the age of 82. In talking to her, I found that she had never had a mammogram. With some prodding, I convinced her that she should have one done.

Surprisingly, the telltale microcalcifications of breast cancer were noted. I scheduled her for a biopsy done with needle localization since there was no lump present. This is done by applying a grid on the mammogram compression plate, taking a picture, and then inserting a needle into the area of the calcifications while the breast is still clamped to the machine. A wire with a barb is inserted through the needle and fixed in the area of the suspicious calcifications. She was then taken to surgery and the area around the wire was excised and a mammogram of the tissue was performed to make sure that all of the microcalcifications were included.

The report came back intraductal carcinoma of the breast. A mastectomy and lymph node dissection was performed and the report returned as no spread or residual cancer found. This was good news. However in December, 1994, five years later, she came in with two superficial lumps just under her clavicle. I removed these two lesions with a generous area of skin and subcutaneous tissue, and the report was high grade ductal breast cancer. This was a discouraging report and I was expecting to see metastases pop up everywhere. Surprisingly, that was the end of the problem, and Wilma finally passed on from natural causes at the age of 92, on November 7, 1999, ten years after her initial surgery.

Mary, age 76, came to see me with a case of bronchitis. As I was listening to her lungs, I told her that I would have to listen to the front of her chest and to her heart. She was somewhat resistant to exposing her chest for the exam, and when I removed her bra, I noticed a large ugly cancer that had eroded through the skin next to the left nipple. I told her that she would need immediate surgery, and I thought that she was somewhat relieved that someone had finally brought into the open what she had been hiding for so long. "Can you really fix me, or am I just wasting your time?" she said. "I never give up hope and neither should you," I said. I did a modified mastectomy and carried the dissection into the axilla and removed all of the visible nodes. Three of these were positive for breast cancer. She healed up without problems but did not want to undergo radiation so she was given Tamoxifen, an anti-estrogen agent as her follow-up treatment.

She developed a pleural effusion and I immediately thought, "Oh, oh, lymphatic spread to the lungs." I put her on a diuretic and a digitalis preparation for her heart after aspirating the fluid, and there was no further recurrence. She was followed regularly but never showed any further sign of cancer and finally moved back to Wyoming with her son at about the age of 84 still free of cancer. She was eternally grateful that I had pressed her into a more complete examination that she was initially not prepared to allow.

The last case is that of Andrew Kindsfater, an elderly gentleman who was in the nursing home when I saw him for a mass in the skin of his lower abdomen. I took Andrew to surgery and removed the mass. The report was metastatic pancreatic cancer.

I went back to his nursing home room when I received the report a few days later and said, "Andrew, I've got some bad news for you. You have pancreatic cancer that has spread, and there is really no treatment available." Andrew looked at me and replied, "Don't worry doctor. An Angel sat on my bed last night and told me that I would be healed." I left his room shaking my head and feeling that he did not understand the seriousness of my words.

I got some blood studies on him so that we could monitor him, and they showed a slightly elevated bilirubin, indicating that his bile ducts were probably starting to get blocked with cancer. His liver enzymes were also slightly elevated. Two weeks later the blood tests were a little better, and he showed no signs of deteriorating health. A month later all the tests were normal, and his wounds from the surgery had healed. Six months later he was in perfect health with no abnormal findings. He died about five years later of natural causes with no signs of cancer at the age of 94.

So, what happened? Did the lab have a foul-up and send the wrong report? Or did an Angel really sit on his bed that night and cure him of his cancer? I am not sure that I have the answer. Do you?

CHAPTER 22
SNAKEBITE

Snakebite is not a big part of any family doctor's practice, but it might be interesting to review the evolving treatment over the years, and to discuss a few of the cases that I have managed during that time frame. Rural Montana is certainly home to its share of rattlesnake bites, but occasionally urban Montana, such as Billings, will report a rattlesnake bite in the back yard of some of the homes that lie under the rims.

When I was in the Boy Scouts, the treatment for snakebite was to make two small cuts in the form of an X over the fang marks and then apply suction. We all had our little snakebite kits that we dutifully carried in our packs as insurance against such an event, but fortunately we never had to use them.

Down in Texas, along the San Jacinto River, we had a scout camp, and we would go on cottonmouth water moccasin expeditions to catch and sell the snakes. We would find them, pin them down with a forked stick, grab them behind the head, and throw them in a burlap sack. The snakes were sold for their venom to a medical facility that used the venom for anticoagulation test kits.

Well, fortunately, no one in our Explorer Scout group was ever bitten, but the treatment of cut and suck is no longer recommended. Likewise, a tight tourniquet to delay the spread of the poison also should not be used. The patient should be kept quiet, and the extremity kept below the level of the heart. Until a few years ago, ice was recommended to keep the extremity cold, with the thought that if it could be kept cold for several days, the poison would break down and dissipate. This also has fallen into disrepute.

Someone came up with the idea of using electricity from a car battery to coagulate the poisonous protein with an electric charge. Wires were placed around the bite areas and connected to the battery terminals and intermittent jolts of electricity passed across the area. This was refined to the use of high voltage, low amperage direct current in a series of small shocks around the bite, and then repeating this in ever widening circles. After anecdotal reports of good results with this technique, a detailed study also put this procedure in the trash bin of antiquity.

The use of cooling and high intravenous doses of corticosteroids also found its way into the medical journals. The theory was that the anti-inflammatory effect of the steroids would keep the swelling and tissue destruction to a minimum until the body detoxified the poison. That seemed to make some sense, and I have used the technique along with intravenous antivenom.

Since horse serum antivenom, and more recently sheep serum anti-venom can sometimes result in a severe allergic reaction, and almost always in delayed serum sickness, steroids are frequently necessary, at least in the aftermath.

So what should be done? First, keep calm and quiet. If you don't have to walk for help, lie down and let someone else go for help. Keep the extremity in a dependent position, and a light tourniquet just tight enough to slow up lymphatic and some venous drainage is in order. Some cooling may slow up the circulation through the area, but packing in ice will injure the tissues. Get to a hospital as soon as possible so that antivenom can be administered.

I remember a young boy about five years old, who was bitten on his hand, and only one fang mark was present. He was playing in the back yard, and the snake was in the flower bed. He must have disturbed it when he went to retrieve his ball. The snake was a small rattler, and at the limit of its strike range, which is about three fourths of its body length. He was brought to the hospital rather quickly, but was already looking pale, with a low blood pressure, and swelling of his hand. We started an IV and administered four bottles of antivenom, which was all we had on hand. His pulse remained good, and he did not develop a compartment syndrome, which occurs when the swelling is so intense that it shuts off the blood supply due to swelling pressure on the veins and arteries. If this happens, the doctor must make an incision lengthwise in the extremity and cut through the fascia overlying the muscle to allow room for the swelling. It can be closed up several days later when the swelling has subsided.

Our little patient made a good recovery, although his hand and arm swelled to the size of his leg before it resolved.

Quentin E was another patient who presented with a snakebite. He was eighteen at the time. The snake hit him twice on the heel and ankle. He got to the hospital within an hour, but the swelling was already starting to get bad, and he was feeling tingling in his face and whole body.

We kept him calm and quiet, and got an IV going. We gave him five vials of antivenom, and then sent a driver to the Crow Agency hospital, twelve miles away for two more vials. He got those about an hour later and began to stabilize. His foot and ankle were huge and eccymotic, (hemorrhages around the wound); but, again, his circulation remained intact with no compartment syndrome, and in three days, the swelling was down enough for him to return home.

The last case was somewhat humorous and the story goes like this. Our softball team was playing a game that we really needed to win. I was our only pitcher that day and a message came from the hospital via the deputy on duty that I was needed at the hospital immediately because one of the Mexican beet laborers had been bitten by a snake and he had passed out prior to getting to the hospital. The softball rules state that if a player leaves the game, and a new inning starts, he cannot reenter the game. I told the team that they would have to try and stay at bat until I had evaluated the patient and then see if I could come back or not.

The hospital was only two blocks away so I got there pretty quickly. According to the patient, he heard the snake rattle, and then the big snake struck him in the leg. He was shaky and weak when he got to the hospital and according to the history, he had fainted. When I examined him, I could find no fang marks and there was no swelling. He was wearing rubber irrigation boots and the snake was unable to penetrate the boot.

It turned out that the rattling was hissing from a large bull snake, and the poor patient got so excited that he passed out from fright, and had no significant injury. I got back to the softball game just as my team made their third out in a long inning of good batting and eight runs, and I was able to stay in the game and resume pitching. We won the game and remained on top in the league standing. Long live the bull snake!

CHAPTER 23
CORONARY CARE

One of the most important advances in medicine during the last fifty years has been in the development of technology to understand and treat heart disease of all kinds. This included congenital problems, valves, and especially the management of acute heart attacks. Prior to the late 1950s, not much could be done for a heart attack except put the patient to bed, give morphine, oxygen, nitroglycerine, and hope for the best.

We had EKG machines that could record the heart beats and print them on a continuous roll of paper. We did not have the monitors for the heart at the patient's bedside that transmitted to a central nurse's station until the mid 1960s, except at some of the large teaching centers. We were just learning that the heart could be defibrillated with paddles and an electric current, but that was usually with the paddles applied directly to the heart after the chest had been opened. Before we had closed chest massage, I remember seeing surgical resident doctors open a chest in the ER and do direct cardiac massage to keep the circulation going to the brain. We actually got to practice this procedure on a dog in physiology class, during medical school.

The heart lung machines were just being developed in the late '50s where extracorporeal circulation could be carried out and the heart beat could be stopped so that the surgeons could operate on the heart more leisurely, and repair defects previously inaccessible when the heart was in motion. The heart could then be opened to repair a valve or close a hole in the atrium or ventricle. We had to make our diagnosis of heart abnormalities by the murmurs heard through our stethoscopes and we spent hours as medical students listening to these murmurs on audiotapes. Later, cardiac ultrasound was developed, and we could get a moving, real time visualization of the blood flowing through the heart and make these diagnoses more accurately.

When a person had a heart attack, the ventricle became irritated electrically, and irregular beats occurred from the damaged area which could cause the heart to go into ventricular fibrillation. Many people died, not from the size of the heart attack, but from the interruption of the normal pumping action of the heart due to the fibrillating, non-contracting ventricle. With the availability of the cardiac monitors, we could now spot these occurrences, and with the availability of a defibrillator, we could shock the heart back to a regular rhythm. This meant that if we could see the abnormal ventricular beats, and especially if there were runs of several together, we could be better prepared to deal with the impending ventricular tachycardia or fibrillation.

This was our scenario in early 1970. If we were to keep our small hospital up-to-date, we had to get a monitor and defibrillator and train the nurses how to use it. I had participated in a continuing education course in December, 1969, and took careful notes on what we all needed to know about how to follow these fresh heart attack victims. Practically no small hospitals in Montana were equipped to deal with this problem at that time. Money was tight for equipment purchases by our hospital, so we needed to start raising funds from the community. I spoke to Tom Sylvester, the hospital administrator at the time, about what kinds of funds the hospital had for the project. He said that we would have to raise all of the funds outside of the hospital's budget. I told him that we really needed a defibrillator so we would get to work on it. I talked to Wally, the Elks Club, and several other people, and we started planning a benefit dance to raise money. We got a generous contribution from J.J. Ping and several others in addition. The dance was a success, raising about $1,500 for a start. Several other organizations, including the hospital auxiliary, also contributed. Before you knew it, we had our monitor and defibrillator machine.

Protocols for closed chest massage and mouth to mouth resuscitation were developed. I put together a course for the nurses on how to recognize the ventricular abnormal beats, including ventricular and atrial tachycardia, ventricular and atrial fibrillation, and the acute changes that were present on the EKG of a fresh infarct. Now, we were ready for our first patient. It didn't take long.

"Sonny" L.H. Hughes presented to the ER in early March, 1970, with severe crushing chest pain. It was obvious that he was having a heart attack, and the EKG showed what appeared to be a large anterior infarct. He was put to bed, given oxygen and morphine, and was hooked up to the cardiac monitor. I had just had my gallbladder removed in Billings two days before and had just returned home, barely able to walk due to the large subcostal incision. In those days, laparascopic cholecystectomy had not been developed, and recuperation from the large painful incision required about three to four weeks. Dr. Carriedo, my partner at the time, was on call, and he had gone grocery shopping at the local Safeway store. Our communications were not as good as today, as pagers had not been available to us. We did have some short range 100 micro-watt walkie-talkies, but he did not take one with him when he went to the store. Sonny began to show some runs of ventricular ectopic beats, and then he went into ventricular fibrillation.

The nurses called the sheriff's department to send someone to the Safeway store to get Dr. Carriedo and they also called my home to see if I could manage to get out of bed to come over. As I was pulling on my pants my wife was yelling at me that I would break open my incision if I tried to get there to help. "I need to get there," I said. The nurses started CPR and fired up the defibrillator. The first shock was at 100 watts and he was still in fibrillation. The power was increased to 200 watts and he was shocked again. The fibrillation stopped and a normal rhythm returned. About that time both Dr. Carriedo and I got there, but the nurses had successfully converted their first patient and prevented the inevitable outcome of losing him, if they not had the new equipment. They were feeling pretty good about the situation, but little did they know that they would have to do it many more times before he could leave the hospital.

We did not know in those days that intravenous Xylocaine, a local anesthetic that we used to anesthetize the skin for laceration repairs, could calm the irritable myocardium, and prevent premature ventricular beats that occurred after a fresh infarct. That knowledge came a few months later. Then, we started using a prophylactic lidoocaine drip after a new heart attack. We had to be careful not to use too much, or we could produce a seizure. We were not out of the "woods" yet with Sonny, and over the course of the next two weeks, we had to defibrillate him about a dozen more times. He was able to leave the hospital after three weeks, and although he had a large infarct that significantly reduced the pumping action of his heart, he lived until February 23, 1978, eight years after his initial heart attack, when he finally passed away from congestive heart failure.

Gertrude Heth was an elderly lady with an enlarged heart and emphysema, whom we admitted for observation for mild chest pain. We had attached her to the monitor. It was surgery day and I was visiting with a post-op surgical patient after she had recovered from the anesthetic. We had moved her post-surgically into Gertrude's room since this was closest to the nurses' station. As I was talking to her with my back to Gertrude, she said, "What's happening to her?" I turned and noted that Gertrude was lying unresponsive on her bed and the monitor showed ventricular fibrillation. I reached up and turned on the defibrillator, smeared on some electrode jelly and applied the paddles. One shock at 200 watts stopped the fibrillation, and after about three seconds of asystole (no heart beat) a normal rhythm resumed. She was not breathing, but after about five minutes of using the bag and mask with 100% oxygen, she resumed spontaneous breathing. She recovered consciousness in about ten minutes. Her EKG did show the findings of an evolving anterior myocardial infarction, but she recovered uneventfully. We asked her if she saw the white light that some people see when they die and are resuscitated, but she didn't. Maybe our prompt intervention had not let her get far enough down the road to see the lights beckoning her onward.

Edna Smith entered the hospital with moderate anterior chest pain. An EKG showed some suspicious changes of a heart attack, but not the typical elevation of the ST segment. We did not have all of the blood enzyme tests at that time that would have helped clinch the diagnosis. We decided to admit her for observation and monitoring. As Lorraine, one of our nurses, was taking the admission information after moving her to the cardiac room, Edna looked up at her and said, "I feel like my heart just stopped!" and then she rolled her eyes upward and fell back on the bed.

I was at the nurse's station writing orders when Lorraine called out "Code Blue." Several of us immediately responded, and started CPR while the electrode leads were being attached to her body. She was in ventricullar fibrillation. We got an IV into her quickly, and I called out "Get me an ampule of bicarbonate." I gave her that and then infused 10 c.c. of dilute epinephrine intravenously into the tubing. By that time the paddles were charged and ready, and I yelled, "Clear." Everyone made sure that they were not touching her as I pressed the button. On the second shock, her rhythm returned to normal and she recovered uneventfully. When she had recovered consciousness she said, "I feel pretty special to have been resurrected from the dead. Thank you so much." All of these patients would surely have died had they not been in the right place at the right time. Our fundraiser and training of the nurses had turned out to be a wonderful success.

The next advance came with the advent of TPA and streptokinase. These drugs, if given early enough, can dissolve the clot that forms in the coronary artery, which then cuts off the blood flow to the myocardium. We had to learn a new protocol again in the evolving treatment of acute myocardial infarction. Waiting an hour to get the patient to Billings after arriving in the Hardin emergency room was not an option that we wanted to accept. We had one of our consultant cardiologists come to the hospital and give us an in-service on how to use the protocol. We were a little on pins and needles the first time we used the TPA. Because It costs $1,500, we had to be sure that the circumstances were right, and that the blood tests and EKG confirmed that the patient was really having an infarct. What a joy it was on that first patient to see the acute changes on the EKG disappear, the crushing chest pain abate as the clot was dissolved, and circulation to the myocardium start to flow again. We would then transfer the patient for further care and evaluation to Billings where, after angiography, either a bypass or an angioplasty would be done. All of these advances in coronary care have to rank as one of the ten greatest medical milestones.

CHAPTER 24
MENINGITIS

Meningitis is a terrible disease, which acts swiftly with devastating results. If treatment is not started soon enough (within a few short hours), death usually results. Meningitis is highly contagious and is for the majority of cases, a bacterial infection. These bacteria usually start their infection in the nose or throat, and then migrate through the veins and lymphatics into the meninges (covering of the brain). There they cause swelling, inflammation, tissue destruction, increased spinal fluid pressure, stiff neck, high fever, coma, and ultimately death.

Before the advent of antibiotics, the death rate was 100%. Two of the most common types of bacteria that cause meningitis are the hemophilus influenza bacteria and the meningicoccus. These bacteria can be present in the normal throat on occasion, and simply be a resident there, living in symbiosis with the other bacteria. The hemophilus bacteria also causes a severe throat infection in children called epiglottis, which can cause the larynx to swell shut causing the child to suffocate.

In the early years of my practice, this was one of the more serious and worrisome problems that I encountered. I spent more than one sleepless night at the bedside of a child wondering if I would have to do an emergency tracheotomy if the breathing suddenly obstructed. Fortunately, we now have a vaccine which is incorporated in the "baby shots" that prevents this horrible disease that occurs both in the throat, ears, and the brain.

I remember several scary, but interesting cases from those early days. What I would have given not to have had to worry over those critical cases!

The first was a set of twins who had been delivered in Billings, since the mother had started her prenatal care there before I arrived in Hardin. They were four months old at that time, and had just been to the pediatrician in Billings for a routine checkup that day. When the mother arrived home, she noticed a reddish discoloration in her son's diaper. She called me to say that she thought it was blood in the diaper. I told her that I would check him to make sure, even though she had just arrived home from the pediatrician. When they arrived in the emergency room with the diaper in question, I immediately noticed that the pink color was actually a precipitate of amorphous urates from the concentrated urine, and that no blood was present. As I was doing this, I had my hand on the baby's head, and I noticed that the soft spot or fontanel was slightly raised. It should have been flat. I sat the baby upright and the fontanel was still bulging. I notice that the baby's skin was warm, and the temperature registered about 100 degrees.

I said to the mother, "The baby's soft spot is bulging indicating that there may be increased spinal fluid pressure that needs to be investigated right now." "Can you do that here? It sounds pretty serious. Have you done a spinal tap on a baby before?" she inquired. "Yes, many times, and I don't think we should wait another minute," I told her. After a little hesitation, she agreed to a spinal tap to check out the problem. I noticed by this time that the baby was fussy and the neck seemed to be a little stiff. The nurse secured the infant on his side, so that he would not move, and I inserted the needle into the spinal canal and let the fluid slowly drip out. I attached a manometer to the needle and, sure enough, the pressure was elevated. As the fluid began to fill the test tube, I noticed that it was cloudy, and not clear, as it was supposed to be. A sure sign of trouble! "I'm pretty sure that your baby has meningitis," I told her as I rushed past her on the way to the lab.

When I got to the lab with the fluid, I centrifuged some of it while saving the rest for our lab technician to do a cell count, sugar, and protein level. These were all consistent with meningitis. The cell button from the test tube was spread out on a glass slide and stained with Gram stain. There, among the white cells, were a few slender rods characteristic of the hemophilus bacteria. A culture was done, but that took several days to complete. I had my diagnosis, though, from the slide, and I began intravenous chloromycetin which was one of the few drugs to which the bacteria was sensitive.

Fortunately, we caught the infection at an early stage, just because the baby had been a little dehydrated and the amorphous urates had precipitated out into the diaper. If we had waited until the next morning for an exam, the outcome might have been different. I asked the mother if the other twin was sick, and she replied no, but she would bring her in the next morning, just to be sure. She again expressed her thanks for my concern about the diaper problem. When the twin sister arrived the next morning, her fontanel was beginning to show increased pressure, and a spinal tap showed that she was just beginning to develop meningitis. She was immediately started on treatment and recovered uneventfully also.

In December 1965, there was an outbreak of meningicoccal meningitis on the reservation. The Crow Indian Hospital was filled with a variety of patients, and they wanted to transfer a very sick patient who was coming in from Lame Deer, Montana, about forty miles northeast of Crow Agency. I did not get much more history, except that his wife was accompanying him in the ambulance. When they arrived, he appeared acutely ill and she said he had become semi-comatose during the ride in from Lame Deer.

His wife said that he was complaining of a severe headache and stiff neck before he became unresponsive. His temperature was 103.5 and his neck was very stiff. "What's wrong with him?" she asked. I was sure that he had meningitis. "I think he has a very bad kind of meningitis from the way he has gotten worse so rapidly. We have to find out quickly and get him on treatment if my suspicions are correct." "Please save him, Doctor, the family needs him so much," she said. I sent the hospital aide for a spinal tray and the nurse and I turned him on his side in preparation for a spinal tap. I scrubbed his back with soap, then alcohol, and inserted the needle in his back. The pressure was elevated and the fluid was cloudy. The centrifuged spinal fluid showed large numbers of white cells, and in the cytoplasm of many were the typical coffee bean shaped diplococci called Neisseria Meningititis. The treatment at that time was sulfadiazine and penicillin. I added some of the aqueous penicillin directly into the spinal canal, and then started an intravenous drip of both penicillin and sulfadiazine. I knew his chance of surviving was not very good. Surprisingly, after twelve hours, he was no worse, and at twenty-four, he was beginning to come out of his coma. Shortly after his admission, his wife started with the same symptoms. We quickly confirmed her disease with a spinal tap and got her on the intravenous antibiotics. Both made a complete recovery.

We were not so lucky with another patient, Frank, age sixteen, who came in comatose. Despite rapid diagnosis and treatment, he succumbed within the first hour of his admission. We had given him mouth to mouth CPR when he stopped breathing. Therefore, all of us had to take oral sulfadiazine for about a week.

We now have a meningicoccal vaccine that we encourage all young people to take before they enter college. Some schools even require it. This has dramatically reduced the rate of meningitis in our young people. Advances in immunization therapy have certainly made childhood and young adulthood a much more pleasant experience, without all of the diseases that my generation had to endure.

CHAPTER 25
THE RESCUE

Almost every vacation that Marlene and I took was associated with a medical meeting and not for just the pure joy of getting away and relaxing. Once, when I started to pitch again after a 20 year hiatus, I noticed that my rise ball just wouldn't move the way it used to do. So I went to San Diego where the "King" or more explicitly, Eddie Feigner, of "The King and his Court," lived. According to many, he was the greatest pitcher ever to pick up a softball. I paid $200.00 for a one hour lesson and picked up a few tips. He may have been the world's greatest pitcher, and he did help me, but my problem as I later figured out on my own, was that I was getting old and my speed had slowed up to the point where the ball just couldn't defy gravity and rise the way it would in days gone past. Well, true to my usual pattern, I combined that pitching lesson with a dermatology seminar, so I could deduct most of the trip anyway.

One year we went to the Bahamas to get some sun and go snorkeling but I got some continuing medical education credits for that one too. One of the few exceptions was when the whole family went to Acapulco, Mexico just to have fun. Fate must have looked down on us and said, "What, no medical meeting?" and promptly hit us with a hurricane that canceled all the swimming, snorkeling, and fishing.

In July 1985, we decided to take a family vacation to the East and see the New England states. We found very little time to really get away as a family with Marlene, Craig, Marc, and myself. Lois was married by that time.

On this occasion we flew to New York City and soon were situated in our hotel. That night we went to the opera **Carmen** and then had cheesecake at Lindy's. No tour of New York City would be complete without a visit to the Empire State Building and a ferry ride to the Statue of Liberty. We visited several historic churches and then the New York Stock Exchange. I finally got to see the place where I was losing all my money. That evening we went to Greenwich Village and saw an off-Broadway play.

I have a friend, Dr. Herb Schaumburg, who is a professor in the neurology department of Albert Einstein Medical College and he lived out on City Island. We made contact and arranged to take the subway out to his neighborhood and then we walked to his home. You remember him in the earlier chapter about polio. He was my scout tent-mate who came down with polio. He managed to pull through despite paralysis and then he went on to great things in medicine. Herb said we were taking our lives in our hands going through the subway routes that were required, but we made it safely to his house. Later, we went out for a fine dinner and reminisced about old times when we were growing up.

The next day we took a commuter airline to Boston and began our tour of Massachusetts. We visited all of the historic sites in Boston, and then rented a car. At Salem we saw a portrayal of the witch trials of the 1700s. We visited the town of Plymouth, and the harbor, where we toured one of the sailing ships, and learned of the hardships that the passengers endured on the long trip to the New World. It must have been a harrowing experience to be cooped up for such a long trip over the ocean. Planning enough food, preserving it, and cooking it must have been a real challenge. Water became foul after a while, so they brought a lot of beer, which stayed drinkable longer, and maybe made the trip a little less worrisome. Then it was a visit to one of the "period" villages, where actors portrayed life in the late 1600s, and it was very enlightening. We learned that dinner forks were not invented until the 1700s. Everyone ate with a knife and a spoon. Forks were for pitching hay.

During all of this fun, I was having an increasingly uneasy feeling that something was just not right with this routine. My life had gotten into a pattern of moving from one crisis to another pretty much non-stop. I had been playing the game of "Doctor, tell me what to do" so long that when I dealt myself out of the game for ten days, I felt lost. Now there was no crisis to solve or problem to handle. I was going into withdrawal like an addict! My addiction was handling crisis and I needed a "**fix**." Then, something happened to change that!

We were all walking on an unpatrolled beach on the coast of Buzzard's Bay when there was a cry of "Help, Help, Help," several times, and it sounded urgent as if someone was in trouble. We looked out in the water, and about 60 yards from the water's edge was a man thrashing and crying out. He was obviously in trouble. He would disappear, then bob up again, and cry out!

I ran to the edge of the water where a small crowd had gathered, but no one was doing anything. One man said, 'I can't swim," and another said "I have a bad heart." I quickly pulled off my shirt, shoes and trousers, (I had my bathing trunks on underneath) and dove into the surf toward the man. At about the same time another younger man dove in along side and we had a race to get to the victim while we could still see him. Evidently, he was wading on a sand bar about sixty yards out where the water was about four feet deep, and the current pushed him off the shallow sand and into some eight foot deep water. He was intermittently going under and then would come up and cry for help. We reached him after our short record breaking race, and each took one of his arms. He tried to clutch at us, so we had to keep him at arm's length until we had him in a firm but safe position and could each grasp an arm and gently swim sidestroke back to the shallow water. I brought him to his wife and briefly checked him over. Although shaken, he was all right. The only casualty was my watch which I had forgotten remove, and the salt water corroded it.

That took care of my feeling of not being needed. Like an addict, I had gotten my "**fix**." The rest of our vacation was uneventful and we toured a few more quaint New England towns before turning in our car and boarding the plane back to Montana.

CHAPTER 26
OBSTETRICS

I wrote about my first C-section in Hardin earlier, and about my training in medical school and afterward. There were some other events that are worth relating, some good and some not so good. Yellowtail Dam was being built when I came to Hardin and there were a number of young families and pregnant women that were glad that they didn't have to make the long trip to Billings for their care. Besides the heavy clinic load, numerous hospital admissions, surgery two days a week, and a busy emergency room, I had approximately 100 deliveries a year.

Dr. Dan Gebhardt was in the Indian Service in Lame Deer in 1972, and I was alone in Hardin. With some help from our senator, we managed to get him out of the two year commitment if he would come to Hardin and join my practice. This was quite a relief for me since now it meant only being on call every other night and weekend.

His wife Patsy was soon pregnant and Dan was hoping for a boy. Patsy was a dedicated runner and was very fastidious about her weight, so she hardly looked pregnant even when she was at term. The day she went in to labor she had done her mile run, having reduced it from two miles the week before.

Everything went smoothly in the delivery room, and soon the baby was crowning and a beautiful baby girl was delivered. I said to Dan, "Well, you didn't get your boy, but you can always try again." Then I noticed that the placenta was not coming down, and when I checked, I felt another baby's head. "Wait a minute, you've got another shot at it, Dan." At that point I delivered a handsome baby boy. Dan and Patsy were as surprised as I was at the twins. We did not have a Doppler to listen to the abdomen for the baby's heart tones in those days, and had to use a stethoscope that fit on the head to give both bone conduction of the heart tones through the doctor's forehead in addition to those conducted directly to the ears. It was called a fetascope. The sounds are not as loud, but I should not have missed the two sets of heart beats.

When Marlene was pregnant with Marc, our second child, shortly after Lois was born, we made arrangements with one of the obstetricians in Billings for her care. His first words were, "Well, since you are a doctor's wife, we can probably expect trouble." That was not exactly comforting and although she continued to see him for the prenatal care, I talked with one of the doctors at the Indian Hospital, Dr. Bunch, who had been helping me with surgery on his days off. He agreed to deliver Marlene at our hospital in Hardin. Her delivery went smoothly and with her saddle block, she delivered spontaneously.

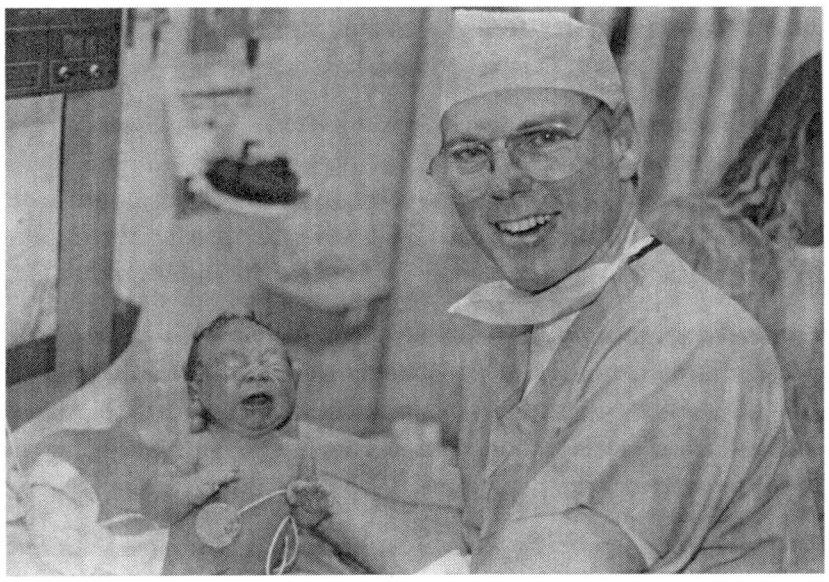

Another one of the many.

It was very difficult to get out of town due to a heavy obstetrical load of about nine patients a month, but finally, after three months of never having left the city limits of Hardin, Marlene and I decided to take the night off, and travel to Billings to see the new science fiction movie, "2001, a Space Odyssey." We had settled in, and were enjoying the movie up to almost the intermission, (it was a long movie if you remember), when a note was flashed on the screen of the movie theater, "Dr. Whiting, please report to the box office." There was a message there to call Hardin, and the report was that one of my patients, Carolyn, a primipara, had entered the hospital in the last stages of her labor. We cut the movie short at that point and rushed back to Hardin, although I knew we would not arrive in time. Terry, one of our more experienced nurses got her into the delivery room, put in some local anesthesia, made an episiotomy and delivered the baby. Everything went smoothly afterward, and when I arrived, I delivered the placenta, and sewed up her episiotomy. Marlene and I saw the last half of the movie ten years later.

At this point, I think I should tell you about some of the various forms of analgesia and anesthesia that were used at the time. When I first arrived in Hardin and began to survey what kinds of equipment, instruments, and drugs that were stocked at the hospital, I found that there was still a bottle of chloroform sitting on the shelf.

Chloroform was first discovered and synthesized by Dr. Samuel Guthrie in 1831 as a substitute for ether. It has a sweet smell and was not explosive, as was ether. Its effect was much more profound, and it attained a moderate following. It was endorsed by Queen Victoria after she used it in her labor and delivery of Prince Leopold. In 1864, it was endorsed by the British Medical Society as Britain's favorite anesthetic. For use in labor, a few drops were inhaled on a sponge with each labor pain and good relief of pain was produced. At that time it was not known that chloroform was broken down into several toxic chemicals in the liver, and damage could occur both to the liver and kidneys. I never used it since it had already been replaced with several other means of analgesia when I began practice. Trilene, or trichloroethylene had replaced it for use in the labor room, and was inhaled through a hand held device by the patient, when the hard contractions occurred. I did use that with fairly good success, but then it was discovered that this compound also caused liver damage. I discontinued its use. Scopolamine was popular with some physicians since it produced amnesia from the painful memories of the labor, but it also caused hallucinations in some patients. I tried it, but quickly discontinued its use. The standard analgesic regime early in the '50s and '60s was Demerol and Phenergan for relief of the pain.

I had good results with hypnosis but not all patients were good candidates, and it did take a lot of the doctor's time during the labor. The La Maz technique of controlled breathing and fixing on breathing instead of the contraction, along with a coach, usually the husband, became extremely popular and we began to give classes in the technique. I still relied on a saddle block type spinal anesthetic at the time of delivery for many of the patients. Later, epidural anesthesia became popular, especially in the larger hospital, but it required an anesthetist to be on site to control the administration of the anesthetic drugs during the labor. Another technique that was more applicable to a small hospital was intraspinal narcotics injected into the spinal canal during labor in tiny amounts which produced good relief of pain for several hours after administration. I found it to be very effective for first time young mothers in labor, but the usage of intraspinal narcotics came much later in my career.

Our third child, Craig, was born in 1968, and he was overdue for several weeks, similar to Lois' birth. Dr. Jim Miech was again practicing in Hardin at that time, and was Marlene's doctor. Her labor was long and hard, and I suggested to Jim that she was probably occiput posterior. At first he didn't feel that that was the case. Finally, he came to the same conclusion, and told the nurse, "Call Dr. Whiting to check her." Sure enough, she was again occiput posterior. We took her into the delivery room and gave her a saddle block. Jim asked me to do the forceps rotation since I had more experience with the use of forceps in difficult deliveries. I put them on and carefully rotated them until the head made the turn. Rechecking the baby's suture lines showed the position now to be occiput anterior. The forceps were removed and reapplied for a standard position. Jim took over and delivered our third and last child, Craig.

Not all things always turn out the way we would like however. I remember two tragic cases in my 2000+ deliveries over the years. The first was a black couple that had been trying to get pregnant for a long time and finally succeeded. The prenatal course was normal and she finally presented in labor. At that time we did not have fetal monitoring, nor a doppler to listen to the baby's heart tones. The fetascope was used to listen to the baby's heart tones. Everything was going well with the last part of the labor when suddenly the nurse noted that there were no heart tones. The protocol was to listen for the heart tones about every five to ten minutes in the last stage of labor. She immediately called me with the report and I got a terrible sinking feeling in my stomach. I rushed over from the clinic, which is only two minutes from the delivery room, and was unable to hear any heart tones either. My patient delivered a stillborn about 15 minutes later. The problem was a short cord with a complete knot in it. When the baby started its decent into the birth canal, due to the short cord, the knot tightened and cut off the blood supply to the baby. Even with current technology, I am not sure that we could have caught the problem in time to do an emergency C-section. What a terrible tragedy for these two expectant parents.

Continuous fetal monitoring was not available at that time. Since then, we have saved many babies who showed signs of fetal distress when this technique finally became state of the art years later. With fetal monitoring, we could tell when the baby was beginning to show fetal distress, with slowing of the heart rate during a contraction. An appropriate C-section could then be performed before the baby was in serious distress. Timing, and the decision whether or not to operate was still a difficult call in many of the cases.

The last case was also very sad. The time was April, 1980. My patient, Eileen, age 32, had a normal prenatal course and finally presented at term in labor. Everything was moving normally as she entered the last part of her labor with good contractions and she was beginning to push. Suddenly she stiffened and then had a seizure followed by unconsciousness. Her right pupil became fully dilated and unresponsive and she stopped breathing. We immediately began bag and mask breathing. Although her color and heart rate remained okay, now both pupils were dilated and fixed. She was essentially brain dead, but we had a live baby still to deal with. By this time the cervix was fully dilated, but the baby's head was still high in the birth canal. I got her onto the delivery table and managed to work the forceps into position and apply traction, working them up and down to gain more leverage. This was a difficult mid-forceps delivery and it required all the skill that I had acquired to that point. Finally, after what seemed to be an eternity, although it was probably no more than three or four minutes, I was able to bring the baby down and complete the delivery.

We were greeted with a weak cry which soon became louder after a little rubbing on the baby's back. I then had the sad duty to relate the incidents to the husband. She had ruptured an aneurysm in her brain with the straining and pushing during the last part of her labor, with enough bleeding in her brain to cut off all of her vital functions. We were still ventilating her with bag and mask, so the next step was to transfer her by ambulance to Billings where they had just installed their new CAT scanner, the first in Montana. We needed to see for sure just what had gone on. It showed a massive subarachnoid brain hemorrhage. After meeting with the Billings neurosurgeon, it was decided to discontinue further life support. It was very sad for her family and me, but we had managed to rescue the infant from a very difficult situation.

There were many other "walking the tightrope" cases during my forty-five years of obstetrics, but fortunately the rest all ended with a happy outcome. We had our share of Down Syndrome patients, cleft lips and palates, club feet infants, and one spinabifida newborn, but these were referred to the specialists in Billings. Neonatal care had now become a specialty; therefore, we had to learn how to catheterize the tiny umbilical veins to get IV fluids and drugs into some of our critical newborns. By that time, we had helicopter service to Billings and could turn their care over to the specialized care personnel. What a relief it was not to have to shoulder all of the responsibility for these cases as I had to do early in my career.

CHAPTER 27
MALPRACTICE

Of all the chapters in this book, this is probably the most difficult to write. No one wants to admit that making a mistake can occur, and it is especially difficult for a physician, since the consequences can be devastating and far reaching. We are frequently put on a pedestal, but we do have feet of clay, just like everyone else. In current day medicine, we are expected to be right with our decision making, technical abilities, and record keeping all of the time. In theory, that should be the case, but mistakes still happen due to a variety of reasons. Frequently malpractice claims arise from either miscommunications or sometimes no communications between doctor and patient. Expectations by the patient and doctor may vary, which is why some consent for treatment forms seem so complicated now. In my early years of practice, we never spelled out all the possible complications. We just said, "Here is your consent for surgery, sign at the bottom." Wow! What a change from now.

In order to help sort out the frivolous lawsuits from the others, Montana has established a medical malpractice panel consisting of three physicians, and three lawyers to hear the complaints and rebuttals. Witnesses may be heard and it is like a mini-trial except that the panel does not have the power to dismiss the complaint. If there is a 6-0 vote in favor of the doctor, it is unlikely that the plaintiff will carry on with the suit. Likewise, if the vote went in favor of the plaintiff, settlement would probably be considered by the physician's malpractice carrier. Judgments that used to be in the thousands are sometimes in the 1-2 million dollar range now, partly accounting for the huge rise in malpractice premiums.

I have had several claims that have gone to the panel and were voted in my favor, and thus no lawsuits were forthcoming, but the worry and strain during those months do take their toll. It hurts when you have done your best, and then you are sued. There were two cases earlier in my career that I am going to discuss in which I had to settle.

In 1962, I had a young couple that came to me for pregnancy who really didn't have much in the way of resources. There was no Medicaid at that time and I guess they didn't qualify for any help from the county. I took care of them and she delivered uneventfully, but they were never able to pay anything on their delivery, so I didn't press them. When the baby was about four months of age I noted that he had an enlarging inguinal hernia, and although I didn't expect to get paid for this either, I agreed to repair the hernia.

On the day of surgery it was cold in the operating room. In order to keep the baby from becoming chilled during the surgery, I told the nurse to fill some hot water bottles and place them around the baby. She did this while I was scrubbing for surgery and the child was anesthetized. The surgery was smooth and uneventful. When I finished the case and removed the drapes, I noticed that the baby had some blisters on his side and thigh obviously caused by the water being too hot. These areas would require dressings and eventually a small skin graft. I told them that I could do the skin graft, but they took the baby to a surgeon in Miles City and brought a lawsuit against me and the hospital. Although I was not really involved in the placing or temperature measuring of the hot water bottles, as "Captain of the Ship," I was responsible for everyone's actions and thus had to settle.

The next case was one in which I certainly learned a lesson in human relations. I had a patient rushed into the clinic with abdominal pain followed by fainting. She was pale, and it didn't take me long to realize that she had a ruptured ectopic pregnancy. She was still bleeding internally. She had been a patient of mine when she was growing up. I had taken out her tonsils when she was younger, and had delivered one or two of her children. We quickly cross matched blood and got her ready for surgery. At surgery her abdomen was filled with blood, and the left tube had ruptured and was still bleeding. I clamped and removed the tube after controlling the bleeding, and removed all of the clots and blood from her abdomen.

We had saved her life and she was now stable. It occurred to me that her husband had scheduled a vasectomy for two days from then. I thought, "If I tie her other tube it will save her husband the risk and expense of surgery, since I would tie the other tube at "no charge." I called him to the operating room door and explained what I thought would be an efficient and economical way of proceeding. He agreed and signed the consent form. Dr. March, one the doctors who worked with me at the clinic, and who was from California, strongly recommended to me that I not do the tubal without her consent, even though her husband had agreed. He said, "people will sue you for anything these days." I said, "John, I've taken care of her since she was little and we have a good relationship. She will thank me for saving them money."

I then proceeded with the tubal ligation on the right side. When she was awake after the surgery, I told her about the ruptured tube, and also that I had tied her other tube in order to save them money on the vasectomy, and prevent the increased risk of her having another tubal pregnancy. I was feeling pretty good about the whole thing and didn't really notice the strange look on her face. Three weeks later I got the complaint from a lawyer that she was suing me for assault and battery. It turned out that she was planning to divorce her husband in the near future, and marry another man with whom she wanted to have more children. Was I blindsided! We had to settle the case out of court. I remember the words that someone once said, "No good deed goes unpunished!"

CHAPTER 28
THE FAMILIES

Neither Marlene nor I came from very large families. I was an only child, and Marlene had one sister. I guess we didn't contribute much to overpopulating the world. We were both depression babies, so our families had to struggle a bit to make ends meet. Since this is about medicine I am going to talk about end of life issues in this chapter.

There is adversity and medical difficulties in almost every family. I think, in retrospect, that we have had our share also.

In February, 1976, an Army recruit at Ft. Dix fell ill, and was dead within 24 hours. Five other recruits were hospitalized, but recovered. Five hundred of the military there tested positive for what was found to be swine flu, a disease usually confined to pigs. With the memory of the 1918 epidemic of influenza still fresh in their minds, the government began a massive campaign to develop and administer a vaccine to forty million people.

The vaccine was ready by October, 1976 and immunizations were hastily begun. On October, 12, it was reported that three elderly people in Pittsburgh were dead within hours of getting the shot. By December, 1976, reports of neurological problems were being reported, especially the rare Guillain Barre syndrome. On December 16, the government suspended the program after having inoculated 40 million people for a flu that never came. By January 1977, more than 50 cases of Guillain Barre syndrome had been reported following the inoculations.

Guillain Barre Syndrome is a form of polyneuritis with symptoms of weakness, primarily in the extremities, and more commonly in males. It usually begins to show recovery within three months of the peak of the illness, but occasionally continues to progress to severe disability or death. It seems to be triggered by some external cause, producing an autoimmune response in many cases, such as the swine flu immunizations.

My father started to notice weakness in his legs several weeks after receiving his immunization, which continued to slowly progress, despite attempts to exercise and strengthen his muscles. At first it was not too bad, and he and my mother went on a three week European vacation in the spring of 1977. When they returned, the weakness was continuing to progress. I flew down to Houston to see him, and I noted the rather profound weakness in both lower extremities. It was apparent that he was not suffering from some nerve impingement or disc disease, and that he was having symptoms of polyneuritis. I knew that reports were now coming in with the same symptoms from people who had recently received the swine flu shot. He progressively became weaker, and the symptoms spread to his arms, and then the muscles of swallowing.

He had expressed to us that he did not want to go on living like this, but we never thought to have this written in a living will. This concept of living wills became popular several years later. His neurologist was unable to make a diagnosis and simply called it a neuromuscular disease of unknown cause. Because of the proximity of the swine flu shot and the onset of his symptoms which somewhat resembled Guillain Barre syndrome, I was sure that he had an unusual form of the disease. Most people recover from this, but a few rare cases had gone on to death. Mother finally had to hire a private duty nurse to care for him at home. Finally, he was unable to swallow, and was transferred to the hospital for care.

He was on IV fluids at that point, and the doctor made a recommendation that a feeding tube be inserted. I could see that the disease was rapidly progressing, and I again flew down to Houston to be with him at the end. It was sad to see this vibrant athlete now wasted to a skeleton struggling for breath. His doctor was reluctant to turn off his IV, so I assumed the responsibility, and wrote the orders in the chart, despite the fact that I wasn't on the hospital staff. I discontinued the IV fluids, and sat by the bed while his life slowly ebbed to a close. I didn't know if he could hear me, but this was a good time to reminisce about things from the past that I had not had time to say. "Dad, do you remember when I first went duck hunting? It was with my Boy Scout troop. You gave me your 12 gauge shotgun to use and we took off early in the morning to the rice paddies near Houston. We were lucky that day and sneaked up on a huge flock of duck as we crawled down a drainage ditch. When our scoutmaster said, "Stand up and fire," it was like World War II. The rice paddy was strewn with ducks. We got our limit that day on the first volley, and then we went into the field to shoot geese. I got a big honker also, and it almost fell on top of me. I was so proud to bring home my limit, and you and I and mother spent the rest of the day plucking them. Then there was all the pitching practice that we did when I first started out. Do you remember all the times in practice that my rise ball was so high that it went over the garage and into the neighbor's back yard? We had to climb over the fence to get the ball. Also, during the games, you would sit behind the home plate bleachers and bawl out the umpire when he wouldn't give me the close ones. There were several times that you had to run out on the field and pop my catcher's dislocated thumb back in place when he caught a pitch wrong. No one seemed to think a doctor was needed and the game just went on. I thought I could see just a hint of a smile on his face as I kept talking. "You showed me how you hit that floater volleyball serve that was so devastating against your opponents when the Houston YMCA won the national championship. You won the last game when your serve just dived away from your opponent and he was unable to return it." His smile seemed to widen just a little, or, it could have just been my imagination. "That was some team that you had in 1938. And how about the fishing that we did when you and Mother came to visit us in White Earth? You couldn't get over the fact that you would get a strike on almost every cast." As I continued to talk about more past events, his breathing began to slow up with longer pauses until it finally stopped. My coach, cheerleader, and father passed away on January 24, 1978.

The other interesting part of this story occurred when I had my friend, Dr. Herb Schaumburg, read the draft of this chapter. I thought my father had died from Guillain Barre syndrome, even though the death certificate read neuromuscular disease and dysphagia of unknown cause. When Herb read the symptoms of progressive weakness beginning in the lower extremities and spreading to generalized weakness, trouble swallowing, and later breathing, muscle cramps, spasms, and fasciculations, he immediately wrote back and said, "Bobby, your father didn't have Guillain Barre syndrome. He had ALS."

How could I have missed that obvious diagnosis? I guess the symptoms following the swine flu shots blinded me to the obvious diagnosis. As for my father's neurologist at the time, he should have picked it up also.

Anterior lateral sclerosis, or better known as Lou Gehrig's disease, is a terrible condition for a person to get. There is no known cure and we really don't know the cause, although about 5% have an abnormal gene leading to some complicated chemistry related to free radicals in the body. It is progressive over one to four years, constantly robbing a person of more and more of his functions on a daily basis, until he is completely paralyzed except for his eyelids and eye movement. The thinking part of his brain remains intact. Feeding tubes and respiratory assistance are required to keep the person alive. Years ago I performed these measures to prolong some of my ALS patients' lives, but for what? I can't imagine living like that. Make sure you have a **LIVING WILL.**

My mother's health had always been good, but in 1955 she perceived what she thought was a small lump in her left breast. She went to our family doctor, but he evidently couldn't feel anything and sent her home. She returned a few weeks later, and he still sent her home with only reassurance. She returned a third time, and at that time he consented to perform a biopsy.

The report was cancer, and Dr, Ehlers, her doctor, followed up the frozen section with a radical mastectomy, in which the breast, the pectoralis major and minor muscles, and all of the lymph notes and fat in the axilla were removed. This was followed up with what was known as super voltage x-ray treatments. It was pretty brutal treatment, and it burned the skin from the radiation. She was cured for 33 years, but I am getting ahead of myself.

In 1985, she went out to get the morning paper and slipped on the icy steps and sustained a rather badly comminuted fracture of her right hip. It was pinned and was slow to heal, so she recuperated at my aunt's home, off Galveston Bay, for about four months before returning home. From that point on, it slowly became apparent that she could not live alone, and my aunt finally called me and said, "Bobby, you've got to come and get your mother. She needs to be with you in Montana." Being home alone in her house with all the memories was not good for her mental health, and I agreed with my aunt. I picked up the phone and called. I said to Mother, "It's time you spent more time with our family and not be alone in your house. It's time for a move to Montana." She was okay with that and soon we packed up her belongings and some of her furniture, and moved her into assisted living at Heritage Acres here in Hardin. It was nice to have her here and there were a lot of people whom she met to keep her occupied. Shortly before the transfer, she had a medical evaluation in Houston, and was pronounced healthy. She came in for a checkup here at the clinic after a few weeks, and was seen by Dr. Greimann, one of my partners. A routine chest x-ray was taken, and as I was passing by the view box, I remarked, "Whose x-ray is that with the big lung cancer?" The nurse said, "That's your mother's."

Evidently the supervoltage radiation treatments used to insure the cure of her breast cancer had, over the course of 33 years, produced a lung cancer. She was worked up by one of the thoracic surgeons, but surgery was deemed not an option. She slowly began to lose ground and finally died on my birthday, November 30, 1988.

Marlene's family also has had its share of medical difficulties. Her father, Tony, called us one day in 1974, saying that he had noted some rectal bleeding, but his local doctor had told him it was just hemorrhoids. I asked him if he had received a proctoscopy, and he said no. At that point in time we did not have our nice flexible scopes, but the standard 25 centimeter rigid scopes gave us a pretty good view of the lower 12 inches of the colon. I told Tony that he should immediately come to Hardin, and I would scope him.

In a couple of days he was here for a visit, and I had him prepped for an exam. At about six inches up the rectum was a large mass which, on biopsy, proved to be cancerous. I took the biopsies, and drove them up to Billings myself, and we got frozen sections immediately. They confirmed my clinical diagnosis. Tony accepted his diagnosis stoically but said that if we couldn't close him up without a colostomy, that he was ready to let nature take its course. I got him scheduled with Dr. John McGahan, and fortunately we were able to do an end to end closure without a colostomy. He healed up fine from that, but a year or two later he developed bilateral inguinal hernias which were repaired by his local doctor. Within a year, they had both recurred. "I seem to be falling apart," he said. Tony returned to Hardin, and I repaired them successfully.

Next, he began to have a few dizzy spells and on checking his pulse, and doing a 24 hour heart monitor test, I noted that he was having significant bradycardia (slow heart beat) to the point of needing a pacemaker. This was put in by the cardiologist in Billings and it successfully corrected the problem. "My Golden Years seem to be collecting a lot of rust on them," he said. Tony had been a smoker all of his life off and on, and now he was getting short of breath. His oximetry reading showed the need for oxygen at night and when exercising. An x-ray showed a suspicious spot at the root of the bronchi, and I sent him to a pulmonary specialist who biopsied the area and found cancer. From that point on, things steadily got worse. Once during the night when he was staying with us, he began to hemorrhage. I felt he would drown in his own blood, but the bleeding finally stopped and he was again stable for awhile. He returned home to Westby for a few weeks, but soon he became weaker. Tony said to his wife, "I think it's time to go to the hospital again." Shortly after arriving, he slipped into a coma and passed away at the age of ninety-one.

Marlene's sister, Sharon, was eight years younger than Marlene and she always depended on Marlene when help was needed. One day in December, 1970, we got a frantic call from her husband. It seemed that they had been to a company Christmas party at K-Mart and were having a good time. Sharon was in her glory. She remarked that the punch was so good that she had five cups of it. At about 4 A.M. she awoke and told her husband that she was hearing voices and that there were snakes crawling everywhere. "What's happening to me," she said.

Her husband, Jim, later found out that the punch had been laced with LSD. He called us, and said, "Sharon's gone crazy." We told him to get her to an emergency room for evaluation.

She was diagnosed as a schizophrenic, but she had no signs of mental problems until the ingestion of the LSD. Jim was unable to manage her or cope with the situation; and, after talking with Marlene, he brought her to Hardin for us to manage. I referred her to Dr. Harr, a Billings psychiatrist. She was initially placed on Thorazine and then other antipsychotic medications, but never really recovered. She returned to Seattle where she felt more at home, but she had a lot of problems, and Jim, her husband divorced her, not being able to cope with the situation. She became an extremely heavy smoker, which led to her untimely death from emphysema at the age of 57.

Dora, Marlene's mother, was the healthy one in the family. She had few problems except for gallstones, and, despite the fact that doctors are not supposed to operate on their own relatives, I took her gallbladder out successfully at her request.

One day, Dora and Marlene were sitting in the kitchen visiting. Marlene was preparing to go to the store, but a phone call delayed her. As she was talking on the phone, she heard a thump behind her. Dora had keeled forward out of the chair and fallen onto the floor. She was not breathing and Marlene could not detect a pulse or heartbeat. She started CPR and called 911 and then the clinic. Dr. Ostahowski, myself and the paramedics all arrived at about the same time. She was in ventricular fibrillation and we asked Marlene if she wanted us to try to resuscitate Dora at her age of ninety-one. Marlene was not ready to let go just yet so she had us defibrillate her heart and continue ventilating her.

There had been some time that she had not been perfusing her brain with oxygen. It left her moderately disoriented following the event and thereafter. We placed her in the nursing home, but she remained confused, and, due to weakness, she would fall. Because of state regulations and "patient rights," we were not allowed to restrain her. Especially at night, she would frequently climb over the bed rails and fall. I had to sew up her head and arm on two occasions. We finally hired an aid to sit with her at night to watch her and prevent the falls. Dora eventually had another cardiac event and passed on peacefully at the age of ninety-two.

I haven't been immune to needing medical care either. Although I have tried to do all the right things such as exercising, maintaining weight, eating right, and watching my cholesterol, things still happen. I was sliding into second base in 1979, and I tore the cartilage in my right knee. This was before the days of arthroscopic surgery, so I had to have the big operation to get to the cartilage. Now, they carefully trim the tear through the arthroscope, and preserve as much cartilage as possible; but then, most of it was taken out on the medial side of my knee. In later life, the joint begins to rub and grind on itself producing arthritic spurs and loose bodies that can get caught in the joint. In November, 1988, I had my knee arthroscoped to trim off the spurs and clean out the joint.

I also had a loose body in the joint which the doctor was unable to find. Shortly afterward, I developed a septic joint with a staph aureus bug and became pretty sick requiring intravenous antibiotics for a few weeks. I was trying to work while taking my three IVs every day. Thankfully, it turned out okay. I was arthroscoped again, and this time the doctor was able to find the loose body and remove it. I already mentioned previously that I had a gallbladder attack in 1970, which required its removal and a few weeks off from work. That was at the same time as our first heart defibrillation attempt using our new cardiac equipment, and with me home from the hospital only three days after surgery.

I have always been able to handle stress on a psychological level, but the body has to respond to it in some manner, which usually means some other bodily system. Evidently, my stomach was the weak link, and I developed a duodenal ulcer that obstructed the outlet of my stomach and required surgery in 1982. The symptoms were really miserable, since the food would collect all day in my stomach and finally pass through the tiny outlet during the night. It was obvious that something had to be done.

The treatment of ulcer disease has dramatically changed in the last fifty years. When I was in medical school, the nonsurgical treatment was a diet consisting mostly of milk and antacids to buffer the stomach and prevent the stomach acids from further eroding the ulcer and causing it to bleed. Sometimes a continuous milk drip given by nasogastric tube was employed. We didn't understand that this just stimulated the stomach to produce more digestive juices and acid as a response. To keep bleeding ulcers or duodenal obstructions from getting worse, more drastic surgical procedures were needed. That was what was recommended in my case. A Bilroth I procedure required slicing open the duodenal bulb lengthwise and sewing it up widthwise to allow free drainage from the stomach into the duodenum. A vagus nerve section is also done to reduce the degree of acid production. There could still be recurrent ulcers and bleeding with this procedure although it was much less formidable than the Bilroth II procedure, which was what my surgeon, Dr. John McGahan recommended. This procedure entailed removal of three-fourths of my stomach and reattachment to a loop of the small bowel ten inches downstream in conjunction with cutting of the vagus nerve. This generally ensures that there will be no further ulcer disease, but the side effects of not much room for food in the stomach, loss of digestive enzymes, and a change in the motility pattern of the entire small bowel are some undesired side effects to live with the rest of a person's life.

In 1983, an Australian doctor discovered, in the lining of the stomach of almost all patients with ulcer disease, a bacteria called Helicobacter pylori. After treatment with antibiotics and eradication of the bacteria, ulcers would heal. This seemed to be the trigger that caused ulcers. It wasn't stress, alcohol, or diet that was the main culprit. Drugs like aspirin, prednisone, and ibuprofin could also cause ulcers, but this organism seemed to be the main player in the puzzle. By this time we had also developed drugs called H2 blockers that would reduce the acidity of the stomach and there was less reliance on multiple doses of antacids to accomplish the task. Then came proton pump inhibitors that would turn off acid production for 24 hours. This drug worked both in ulcer disease, in gastritis, and more importantly, in acid reflux disease that erodes the esophagus causing strictures, inflammation, and sometimes cancer. Ulcer surgery has now become a rare option instead of the main treatment for recurrent ulcers.

My last medical incident to relate occurred on a skiing trip. In February, 1980, our local ski club took a trip to Big Mountain in Whitefish for few days of great skiing. I had skied there before when I had attended medical meetings on the mountain, and was leading our group down the ski slope when we got to a small stretch of snow covered road where the grooming machines traveled. Somehow, one of my skis hit a clump of ice and the ski turned slightly outward so that my skis were getting progressively farther apart and I couldn't un-weight one to correct the problem. Although I wasn't going fast, I finally had to crash straight forward with my skis wide apart. I heard a loud pop in my left knee that sounded like a gun going off when I hit the snow, and I knew that something pretty bad had happened. I had torn my medial collateral ligament and anterior cruciate ligament, and my knee was completely unstable. That ended the ski trip for Marlene and me. We caught the plane back to Billings the next day for me to undergo open surgical repair. The surgery went okay, but my wife kept bugging the nurse that my toes were turning blue and the cast was too tight. I was a little too "out of it" with the post- op narcotics, but fortunately my wife could recognize that the cast had to be split. Finally, the nurse on duty got two orderlies to come up to my room with a cast saw but neither of them had ever split a cast before. By that time I was awake enough to show them how to hold the saw so that it wouldn't cut too deeply, and with my careful supervision, we got the cast split and the pressure relieved. My toes resumed their pink color.

Well, now I was on crutches, which made working and standing without weight bearing a little difficult. It also created a rather unique delivery story. I had an obstetrical patient that was at term, and was scheduled for a repeat C-section. I really didn't want to send her to Billings, so we worked out a plan in the O.R. The nurses got me a dress, since I couldn't get scrub pants over the non- weight bearing cast. They placed sterile drapes on a walker next to the operating table. One of the nurses said, "With a little lipstick and a wig, we could probably get you a date." I did the C-section standing on one leg with a few short pauses to use the sterile walker for a rest. I think that might have been frowned on in a large hospital, but what the heck! I worked fast, the surgery went smoothly, and the mother was happy to remain at home in Hardin.

About that same time Jack Wiechman, a local business man, was starting a ham radio operator's course as part of the evening adult education program at the high school. I could do the classwork and the homework sitting down so that filled some of my healing time. I had always wanted to learn about being a ham radio operator. I took advantage of this time to learn the material and I   got my ham license. There was a lot of math, physics, and also memorization of many rules and facts in the course. I had to bring back to mind my college physics concerning amperes, volts, ohms, resistance, and harmonics. Learning the Morse code alphabet was also required. Now I could communicate with people all over the country, and sometimes the world, via Morse code. What fun!

Our children also had their medical situations to deal with. Lois, our daughter, had urinary tract infections when she was three, associated with reflux of the urine up into the kidneys. We took her to one of the urologists in Billings, and he scheduled her for cystoscopy. I was there during the procedure and was pretty alarmed by the anesthesiologist's failure to monitor her heart when he was anesthetizing her with the Vinethane drip ether. I have seen the heart almost stop with too much, too fast. Then during the procedure, the light on the cystoscope burned out and they didn't have another one to use. Fortunately, the urologist was near the end of the procedure, so it was terminated. He told us that due to the reflux, he wanted to reimplant her ureters into the bladder which was a popular fad at the time. At the termination of the cystoscopy, he used a urethratome, which slices open the urethral opening, and theoretically reduces further infections. Two days later, she began to hemorrhage from the procedure to the point that we had to take her to our hospital and transfuse her. I was really worried about the situation. When it's just a patient, it's easy to do the right thing, but when it's your own flesh and blood lying there bleeding, things are scary. The bleeding finally stopped after irrigating the clots from her bladder and inserting a large catheter. It was pretty nerve-racking. We took her to a pediatric urologist in Houston for another opinion regarding the reimplantation procedure, and also for a visit with my parents. The specialist there said that almost all young children will reflux for several months after severe urinary tract infections. All we had to do was to keep her on antibiotics for several months and then re x-ray her. After this treatment, the reflux had disappeared and she had no further significant problems.

My last family anecdote is about our son Marc. He developed a hernia when he was a few months old, so I had one of my surgeon friends in Billings repair it. The infant hernias are easy to fix, since no strengthening procedures are needed. The hernia sac has to be carefully dissected from the cord, and then a high ligation of the sac is done and the operation is over. Since babies are so small, and the structures are tiny, the surgery is a little more delicate than on adults. I had scrubbed in on the surgery, and told Marlene afterward that everything went OK. We waited for Marc to be brought down from the recovery room, but after about an hour we were getting a little concerned that he had not been brought back to his room. I called up to the recovery room and they said that no one was there. They had temporarily lost him! Finally, one of the cleaning ladies heard a baby crying in one of the utility rooms, and it was Marc. Evidently there had been some sort of emergency in the recovery room and Marc had been moved out of the way so they could attend to the problem. No one acknowledged how he was left there unattended. I wish we had kept him in our local hospital for surgery where nothing like that can happen!

CHAPTER 29
THE DOCTORS

Those readers who don't live in Big Horn County might find this chapter one that they can skip, but for history's sake, I felt it needed to be included. When I began researching the records of the hospital regarding the different doctors and their time line, I thought for sure that the records would be easy to find, but that wasn't the case. There was no credentialing file. Also, the State Board licensing records do not go back past ten years, and the local newspaper was pretty devoid of news stories too. This required a lot of head scratching and asking around, since all the records at the Hardin Clinic that were older than ten years were also destroyed unless the charts had remained active.

When I got to Hardin, Dr. McFarland was still practicing, but he was in poor health, and he retired in 1962. That left me alone in Hardin, with a busy practice, no time off, and emergency room calls every night. Sleep was at a premium.

Since my residency, Marlene and I had kept in contact with Jim and Marilyn Miech. Jim and I were both residents at Monterey County Hospital and had become friends during our time there. Jim was finishing his two year military commitment with the Coast Guard in 1963 and now needed to look for a place to practice. His parents lived in Sheridan, Wyoming, only an 80 mile trip south, and they were getting a little older, so that being close to them was a good selling point. Jim accepted my offer and joined the practice. Now, I could have every other night and weekend off. The practice was busy and growing during that year, but Jim got an offer from a clinic in Alameda, California, with more time off, and not such a hectic schedule as we had in Hardin. After one year in Hardin, Jim, Marilyn, and Stevie, their son whom I had delivered during that year, moved back to California. Alone again!

I heard that John Iwakiri, a local Hardin boy, was finishing his internship in Portland, Oregon. His parents were elderly and needed some looking after, so I flew to Portland, and met with him to present a proposal to practice with me in Hardin. He was agreeable, and as soon as his internship ended, he moved back to Hardin. John was a good doctor, but after three years, I think he felt that family practice was too encompassing and demanding for a lifetime career. He had always been interested in ophthalmology, and in the summer of 1967 he left for a residency position in this specialty. It was back to the drawing board again.

As luck would have it, Jim Miech had not found the position in California just what he wanted, so he moved back to Hardin, but this time in his own separate practice. Almost at the same time, another doctor, Travis Hindman, came through Hardin and decided to set up a separate practice here. There were now three of us in separate practices but we were able to work out a call schedule for the ER, and also assist could assist each other with surgery and anesthesia. Then the proverbial fly flew into the ointment. This was now 1968. Things were going great, but nothing stays the same forever, as I had already noted with our doctor situation. My wife was working at the clinic one day and a call came in from Dr. Hindman's secretary asking if I could see his patients as he had gone to Billings. My wife asked when he would return. After a pause, the answer was "never." He and his wife divorced shortly afterward and he eventually went back into a residency and became a pathologist. At the same time Jim received an excellent offer from a multi-doctor clinic in Menomonee, Wisconsin. In December, 1968, he closed his practice in Hardin. This left me alone again.

Dr. "Hermy" Cabrerra was practicing in Worden, Montana, just east of Billings, and north of Hardin, and he had invited a colleague, Dr. Rodolfo Carrieido, to join him. There were not enough patients for a two man practice there, and Dr. Carriedo decided to move to Hardin in 1969, and join the practice here. He stayed for two years, but then in 1971, he took a position with the VA as a staff physician.

Several members of the Chamber of Commerce helped form a committee to look for a doctor for Hardin, and we heard that Dr. Dan Gebhardt was practicing in the Indian Service in Lame Deer, but was not really happy there. This was his military commitment. With the help of our senator, we were able to have him finish his service time as a member of the Hardin Clinic, since we were an underserved rural area. He joined the practice in 1972. Dan was well liked by the staff and the community in general, but after two years, and finishing his military commitment, Dan decided to move back to his home state of Oregon, and join a larger practice with more time for his family and himself.

To alleviate the physician shortage in rural areas, several states had initiated physician assistant programs for problems of a less complicated nature, which would give physicians in these underserved areas a little respite. Montana had no legislation or physician assistant program at that time, but I knew that the University of Salt Lake had a program to train people for this type of work. They had to have previous medical experience, such as military corpsmen, ambulance personnel, or nurses. The Nurses' national group was also beginning to develop their own program for registered nurses to undergo additional training and practice independently from the doctors as Family Nurse Practitioners. Physician Assistants practiced under the supervision of physicians. The Salt Lake program required previous experience to enter, then, a one year lecture and lab program, followed by a one year preceptorship with an approved physician. I went to Salt Lake, met with the director of the program, and also with a promising student, Rick Schurman. I was appointed assistant professor of medicine on their staff in order to be a preceptor. Rick was just finishing his classroom year at that time. Soon, he was headed to Hardin. He had been a Navy Corpsman, had worked for an ENT doctor, and also for an orthopedist, so he brought those skills to the practice. To complete the program, each student had to see and treat at least three each of a variety of medical, surgical, pediatric, dermatologic, and gynecologic conditions and have these charts reviewed in Salt Lake City. All of his day to day charts had to be reviewed by me for history, physical findings, treatment plan, and differential diagnosis.

We still had no physician's assistant legislation on the books in Montana, so I had to get a bill drafted and get someone to sponsor it in the legislature. The Nurses' Association lobby was strong in Montana, and they had their lobby personnel work hard against it. I felt like a lone voice in the wilderness, and speaking before a Senate committee to plead my case was not what I went to medical school to do. I explained that Montana had many small towns with only one doctor, and that we would die on the vine if we didn't get some relief. Small town hospitals cannot function without a physician, and most physicians would not want to practice in a town without a hospital, so we had to succeed. We finally got a watered down version passed which said that all charts had to be reviewed daily, and all prescriptions countersigned by the physician. This really defeated the purpose of a physician assistant, which was not only to help lighten the load on the physician, but also to allow him to have a weekend off occasionally. It was a small step, but it was better than nothing.

Rick got married during his time in Hardin, and in 1975 he and his wife moved to Portland. He was working for an ambulance company there as a paramedic, and an interesting story occurred as a result. One of our nurses in Hardin, Lorraine Kuntz, had a twin sister, also a nurse, who worked in one of the hospitals in Portland. One evening Rick was on ambulance call and had to deliver a baby in route to the hospital. Lorraine's sister was called down from the maternity floor to help with the busy ER as Rick came through the door with the newborn and mother. He spied her and said, "Well, hello Lorraine, what are you doing here?" When she didn't seem to recognize him, he said, "Don't you remember when we were working together in surgery at Hardin?" She replied, "You must mean my twin sister, Lorraine." Rick had a hard time believing that she was not putting him on, but they finally had a good laugh about it.

It was discouraging to keep having doctors move away to greener pastures. My wife kept asking me why we didn't also move where I would not have to be on call continuously and in the emergency room almost every night. I had to keep telling myself that if I left, the hospital and nursing home would close, people would be out of work, and there would be no one to handle all of the emergencies and serious problems that happened on a day to day, or even an hour to hour basis. Once a hospital closes, it is very difficult to get it open again. "Things had to get better if I could just hold out a little longer," I thought to myself.

Our physician recruitment committee became active again, and a National Health Service site was created after jumping through a few government hoops. Clint Moen was recruited in 1975 and the NHS rented space from the clinic. Clint did a good job, but after a year Clint and his wife divorced and toward the end of 1976, he left. Dan Gebhardt returned for 2 years in 1976 in a separated practice and was also doing Locum Tenems around the state, since by now he had become a pilot. The NHS recruited Bob Arfman in 1978 and Steve Hubbard was added in 1979. The three of us practiced at the Hardin Clinic until 1981 when the site was dissolved. I obtained another physician assistant, Tim Saunders in 1979 and he stayed until 1982. Shortly afterward, Steve Wolk, another physician assistant joined our practice.

The committee recruited another physician, John March, to join me in August, 1981, and he brought additional skills of laparoscopic pelvic surgery to the clinic. John had gone to school at Berkley, University of California, during the flamboyant seventies, and he brought a different perspective to rural Montana. He and his wife were Quakers, vegetarians, and had a deep feeling against violence and war. He broadened the scope of the types of patients that we saw in the practice. Dr. Gary Ostahowski had been in the Indian Health Service at Crow Agency for several years and decided to join Dr. Gebhardt's practice in 1981. In June, 1983, Gary joined our practice and we formed a partnership which consisted of the three of us, John, Gary, and me. Dan moved to Spearfish in 1984 to open a clinic there, and to offer chelation therapy to a large group of patients seeking that type of therapy, in addition to regular family practice.

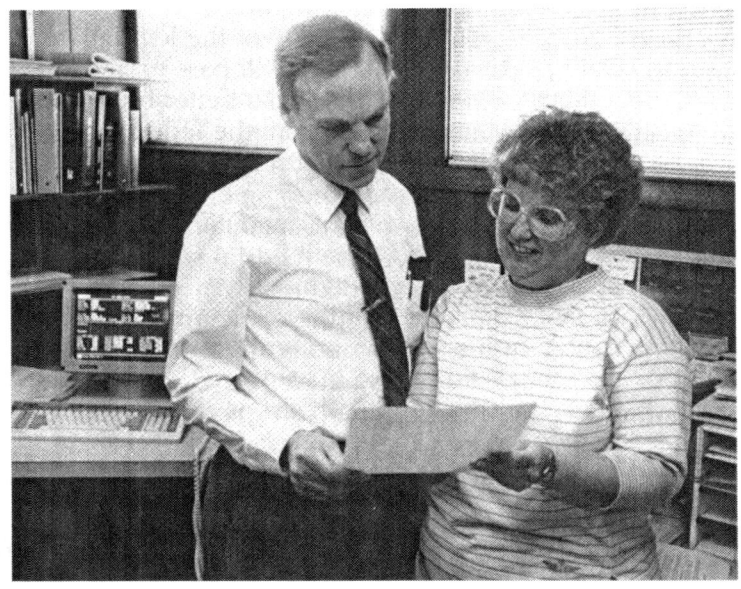

Keeping records at the clinic with Glennine Schoen in 1989.

Dr. Carol Greimann and her husband, Gene, a veterinarian, were exploring Montana for a place to open both of their practices, and they visited Big Horn County in August 1984. Carol had a commitment to the NHS for four years of service and she interviewed at Crow Agency as a potential site. She also paid us a visit since we were still considered a medically under served community, and liked what she saw. She joined our partnership, and Gene opened a veterinary practice also. We were all very busy and the practice flourished. At about this time, John had a foot injury that precluded him from being able to stand for long periods which is what doctors have to do, either in surgery or just as an average day requires. John was always interested in psychiatry, and he entered a residency in Durham, North Carolina, and has since become a rather renowned child psychiatrist there.

In 1990, Kim Caprata, a nurse who was working at the Lame Deer PHS facility went into the Physician's Assistant Program at Grand Forks, N.D. The Hardin Clinic agreed to sponsor her for the clinical part of her preceptorship. When Kim finished her training and became licensed as a Physician Assistant, she went to work for the Hardin Clinic and remained as one of our long term staff. This was one of our better decisions, since Kim has been with the clinic for 18 years.

We added another doctor, Bill Beatty, who stayed for about a year before he and his wife moved to Helena, their home town. The clinic was now bulging at the seams and medicine had become much more complicated from a business point of view. We added another doctor, Sam Artzis to our group at about that time, and patient room space began to be at a premium. Sam was offered the opportunity to take over the practice of a retiring physician in the northern part of the state, and the offer was too good to turn down. Reluctantly, he moved. Carol, Gary, and I felt that if we were to grow and offer more services, we would have to have more space. A plan was developed to build a new clinic that the County would own, and we would rent. We would give our current Hardin Clinic building to the Hospital Association for a charitable gift. We sold our assets and equipment to St Vincents hospital and became paid employees of their network. This got rid of the problem of negotiating with various insurance groups, HMOs, PPOs, and government agencies. I had now been full circle from working for a hospital as an intern to working for a hospital as a staff doctor.

CHAPTER 30
ORTHOPEDICS

Orthopedics has always been a considerable part of Family Practice for those doctors in this specialty who spent enough extra time and effort to handle the routine fractures and sprains that occurred almost daily in the course of a busy family practice. The key is, that in order to be good at something, one needs to do it frequently, until it almost becomes routine. When I was in the Indian Service, my partner, Roy Wittwer, had a lot of family practice orthopedics training in the first year of his residency, and on the Indian reservation, there were plenty of injuries, accidents, and trauma to present us with considerable exposure in treating these injuries. I rapidly learned under his tutelage how to put in a local block for a fractured forearm, bend the distal part almost to a right angle, apply traction, and with my thumb, shove the distal part forward enough to slip it over the fracture site and fall into place. When both the radius and the ulna were fractured, it became little more difficult to get them both reduced at the same time, but with a little practice, I became quite good at it. We cared for a large variety of simple fractures, and even a few compound or open fractures with good results.

When I entered my residency, I had enough experience to handle most of these without calling in the consultant for help. I did learn about a rather common problem to which I had never been exposed, from one of the other residents, Myron Gananian. This was "nursemaid's elbow." This injury occurs when an adult is lifting a young child by the arm over an obstacle such as a curb. The proximal end of the radius dislocates and the child will not use his arm although it looks perfectly normal, as does the x-ray. With a simple maneuver of pressure over the radial head at the elbow and a quick pronation of the child's forearm, a click is felt under the doctor's thumb, and suddenly the child is cured. It looks like a miracle to the parent. I have treated so many of these over the years, and have received a lot of thanks by the parents for my recognition and treatment of the problem.

When I arrived in Hardin, I found a consultant in orthopedics, Dr. Perry Berg, who was an enormous help in furthering my education. Every Thursday afternoon I would travel to Billings and bring with me all the charts and x-rays of the fracture cases that I had treated for the week. I would show him the x-rays, and discuss the treatment plans. This kept most of the patients from having to make a trip to Billings; of course, Dr. Berg got all of my complicated referrals. He gave me confidence in handling cases that I might not have wanted to treat without his assurance that I could manage them.

My patients also seemed to have confidence that I could handle most of their problems. This brings up an interesting story about young Doug Freeman. His father, Doug senior, was a lawyer, and played with me in the Dixiland band. Young Doug fractured his femur in a snowmobile accident and was brought into Billings where he was seen in the ER. The family was told that he would have to be in traction for a considerable time, and the doctors there recommended that the family continue on to Hardin for me to care for his fracture. It was later in the evening by the time he arrived, and it was obvious that he would have to be placed in what is known as balanced traction to stabilize the fracture. This required a hospital stay of about three weeks before the fracture was "sticky" enough for him to be placed in a body cast. In order to set up the balanced traction I had to drill a pin through Doug's knee area so that the attachments and weights could be applied. I decided to save money by doing this in the patient's room instead of the operating room or ER, but I needed an assistant. The nurse was partly occupied with other duties so I told Doug senior, "You'll have to be my assistant and help me by holding his upper leg steady when I drill through the bone." I gave young Doug a sedative, placed the sterile drapes around the working area and put in a local anesthetic where I would be drilling. Doug senior steadied the leg, and I became intently occupied in drilling the Kirshner wire pin through the bone. I heard a "clunk" and looked up to find that Doug senior had become faint and had fallen to the floor. By that time, I had finished the drilling so the nurse and I attended to Doug senior. He rapidly recovered, and I then hooked up the traction weights to the pin that I had drilled through the knee. Doug junior had a normal course of healing, and in about three weeks we put him in a body cast called a hip spika and sent him home to continue his healing. The moral of the story is that if you include the lawyer as your surgical assistant, you won't be sued.

One of the scarier stories involved my daughter, Lois. We had gone skiing at Antelope Butte, near Sheridan, Wyoming, one Sunday. As Marlene and I were going up the upper rope tow, we heard a voice crying out from the lower tow, " I broke it, I broke it." Recognizing Lois's voice, we quickly skied back down the mountain to where she had fallen. We moved her into the infirmary and I examined her leg. It was obvious that she had had sustained a spiral fracture of her tibia, the main weight bearing bone of the lower leg. My plan was to put her in the back of our station wagon, drive back to Hardin, and cast the fracture with a long leg cast. By this time it was beginning to be dusk, and we had about 75 miles to go before arriving in Hardin. About halfway home, I looked at the gas gauge of the car, and we were almost on empty, with not enough gas to make it all the way to Hardin. By this time it was dark, cold, Sunday night, and a long way to go with an almost empty gas tank. We limped into Lodge Grass on "fumes" only to find that the only gas station was closed. What a dilemma! They usually roll up the sidewalks by six o'clock, but we found one person who knew the name of the man who owned the station, and fortunately he was home. He came down and opened up so that we could fill up and continue our trip into Hardin. The rest was routine, and after x-raying Lois's leg, I put on a long leg cast and took her home to recuperate. She was on crutches for about eight weeks, but healed without any problems and was able to resume her dance lessons after about three months. The story reminds us that in the winter one should always have a full tank of gas, a coffee can with a candle, matches, jumper cables, gloves, and a blanket for emergencies.

Another orthopedic procedure that I felt I had to learn was carpal tunnel surgery. For some reason, that had been lacking in my training. I had never heard lectures about it in medical school, and had never seen a case in internship, Indian Health Service, or residency. Now suddenly, in practice I began coming across patients with painful hands at night, and with the numbness and pain in the distribution of the median nerve at the wrist. The reason for my lack of knowledge was that it wasn't a common problem when I was undergoing training. This term was first used in the literature in 1938, but the pathology was not really identified until the 1950s and '60s when it was described by Dr. George Phalen of the Cleveland Clinic. It wasn't prevalent until the 1990s when larger numbers of workers became afflicted from work related repetitive injuries using computers and various other machines. Cashiers, checkout clerks, assembly line workers, and secretaries all can get this condition when either hand position, or repetitive trauma causes the tendons to swell or become inflamed, putting pressure on the median nerve due to lack of space. In fact, almost every profession has certain activities inherent in the job that can cause symptoms.

I remember one patient who developed it working in a meat preparation establishment in which her job all day long was taking a meat cleaver to chop up the chickens. It resolved with a change of jobs. Sometimes that is not an option, and surgery may be required if night splints to prevent flexing of the wrist during sleep, or an injection of cortisone into the canal does not resolve the problem.

In any event, the condition occurs when there is not enough room for the median nerve and nine flexor tendons to pass through a small tunnel in the wrist which is covered with a thick ligament that forms its upper boundary. The operation is not difficult, just delicate. Since Dr. Berg's group included a hand surgeon, I asked him if I could come to Billings and scrub in on the cases that I referred and any other ones that he was doing. Dr. Tom Johnson, the hand surgeon, was a wonderful teacher and was glad to teach me the procedure. After helping with four cases I believed that I was ready to perform the procedure. In a small hospital the requirements for performing procedures were not spelled out in those early years; therefore, when I thought that I was ready to add a new operation to my repertoire, I just did it. Now, because of more insurance regulations, hospital policies and other government supervision, a non-specialist would probably have to perform a much larger number under supervision before he could be allowed to add a procedure to his list of operations.

I read about a new technique called an intravenous lidocaine block for producing anesthesia for any hand or arm surgery at about the same time. I was good at doing regional blocks, but this was much simpler. Since the carpal tunnel operation was done using a tourniquet to prevent leakage of blood into the area which could obscure visualization of the delicate structures, all that was needed was to start an IV in the hand, apply a tight bandage to squeeze out all the blood in the lower arm, pump up the blood pressure cuff to keep any blood from entering the arm, remove the elastic bandage, and fill the veins with 50 cc of dilute lidocaine. Complete anesthesia ensues and lasts until the tourniquet is deflated.

I was now ready to do my first carpal tunnel operation. The patient's symptoms had been present for a number of months and she was already beginning to show a little muscle atrophy from the constant pressure on the median nerve. I put in the anesthetic solution and got good loss of sensation throughout the hand and forearm. "Wow," she said. "I can't feel a thing. Have you started yet?" Her hand was scrubbed and sterile drapes were applied. I made an incision following the linear crease in the palm and extended it proximally to just before the transverse crease at the wrist. I carefully deepened the incision down to the carpal ligament, and slowly divided this thick ligament. "Things are going great," I said to her. I inserted a small self retaining retractor and spread it apart. There beneath the cut ligament was the gray median nerve. I could see an indentation or "hour glass" compression where the carpal ligament had pressed. The operation was certainly indicated. I freed up the nerve and made sure there were no other areas of compression. I then closed up the wound and applied a dressing and splint. "Well, we're done. How do you feel?" I asked. "I'll let you know when the life comes back in my fingers," she replied. As soon as the anesthesia had worn off, she noticed that the constant pain that she had experienced was gone. She healed up beautifully and was a very thankful patient. Since she had been plagued with this condition a long time before seeking help, all of the atrophy did not resolve, but this nice lady had no further pain. This is a very rewarding procedure for those patients where night splints, cortisone shots, or a change in activities does not help. Since that time, carpal tunnel surgery has been another procedure that remained in Hardin and did not have to be referred to Billings.

There was another procedure with comminuted wrist fractures that I performed that has now been replaced with a device called an external fixator. Frequently an elderly patient would fall on her wrist and it would be broken into several pieces. Despite getting the fracture anatomically reduced, it would not stay that way due to the pull of the muscles. After a week when the patient returned for an x-ray, the fragments would be pushed outward and the forearm shortened toward the radial side. In order to prevent this, one would have to drill a pin through several of the metacarpals and another pin into the fractured radius proximal to the fracture. Then, after getting a good reduction of the fracture, one would incorporate the protruding ends of the pins in the cast to prevent retraction from occurring. Today, with the use of the external fixator, the fracture can be "fine tuned" by lengthening the distance between the pins with the use of a screw like device, and even the angle of the pins could be changed. After a few weeks, when the fragments have begun to heal in place, the fracture could just be casted.

I continued to learn more orthopedic procedures, including open reductions and the use of plates and screws. As malpractice cases became more common in general, if a perfect result could not be obtained, I decided to refer those cases to my orthopedic consultants and avoid any possible malpractice risks. Orthopedics was still one of my most favorite activities. Marlene asked me why I didn't just go back and take a residency in orthopedics; but after all is said and done, nothing beats Family Practice.

CHAPTER 31
SURGERY

Although there have been a lot of extremely interesting medical cases throughout the years, the surgical ones seem to be the cases that stand out the clearest in my memory.

Montana cowboys are tough, especially bull riders. I recall shortly after having arrived in Hardin, a bull rider was brought in during a local rodeo. He had been thrown and then trampled by the bull and it was obvious that he had multiple broken ribs. It was getting harder for him to breathe as the minutes went by and an x-ray showed that in addition to multiple rib fractures, he had bilateral collapsed lungs where the ribs had punctured the lungs and allowed air to escape into chest cavity making it progressively more difficult to expand the lungs. He needed chest tubes on both sides to suck out the trapped air and expand his lungs or he would suffocate and die. At that time we did not have the nice chest tube kits that we have now with the chest tube trocars, fluid bags pre-filled with colored water to just the right levels, and all of the instructions written down so that it could be put together quickly.

In my training I had never put in chest tubes and we did not have a setup immediately at hand. I had to find some sterile tubing of the correct size, cut it at a slight angle so that it had somewhat of a beveled end, get some gallon jugs with two hole stoppers, cut some glass tubing to fit the holes and some connectors to attach between the improvised chest tube and the underwater seal. This would prevent excessive intra-thorax pressure from building up but we needed some negative pressure in the bottles. This required a water jug with a three holed stopper and tubing attached to a suction pump. The desired negative pressure could be obtained by the amount of water in the jug with glass tubing in the third hole under the water level. If the negative pressure was too high, it would suck in air through the submerged glass tube and keep the pressure just right.

Now I was ready for the patient. I made a small incision in the chest wall under local anesthesia, spread the intercostal muscles between the ribs with a clamp, punctured the pleura with a clamp and shoved the tube in several inches. A few sutures in the skin which were tied to the tube finished the job. I attached the tubing to the suction apparatus and repeated it on the other side. His breathing was much improved and he would no longer be in danger of suffocating. He whispered to me in a muffled voice, "Thanks Doc, but I have a question. When can I start riding the bulls again?"

Over the years I was able to add surgical procedures to my repertoire, both by study, workshops, and by scrubbing in with doctors, and observing their techniques. I was comfortable with performing abdominal hysterectomies, but had never done a vaginal hysterectomy. I had learned the other vaginal procedures of cystocele and rectocele repair for fallen bladders and incontinence, and how to excise a Bartholin cyst from the pelvic area. I was able to tighten up the pelvic structures that had become relaxed after multiple deliveries, but sometimes the uterus was literally falling out.

I was in Houston visiting my parents and doing continuing medical education, (CME), so I arranged to go into the OR at Methodist Hospital and observe one the gynecologists who was especially good at vaginal hysterectomies. He was very accommodative to my request to observe his technique, and he taught me a great deal in a short time from watching him operate. He made it look easy when he did it, but when I did my first one, it took much longer.

My first patient was an elderly lady with a uterus that would literally pop out with straining or standing. She had to wear a pessary in the vagina to keep it in place, but that was quite a nuisance for her. Because she was elderly, the uterus was small, and bleeding less of a problem, so she was an ideal candidate for my first case. The procedure is not difficult provided one understands the anatomy and can get good exposure, as the clamping, cutting, and tying takes place. The problem that can occur is if a clamp slips, or a suture breaks, when being tied. A bleeder can then retract upward out of the field and it becomes difficult to find it again. An ounce of prevention is worth a pound of cure. The operation went smoothly, and after the uterus was out, I was able to repair her prolapsing bladder and cure her urinary incontinence. She was a happy lady, and was out of the hospital in a few short days, instead of a longer period that would occur if an abdominal incision was required.

Hernia repair was initially a complicated procedure when doctors first started learning how to repair the groin defects. Failures were more common than successes and deaths would frequently occur. There were many techniques employed named by the different doctors who invented them, and most fell by the wayside as better methods would be developed. I remember buying a book about 300 pages in length, just on the repair of hernias. The trick was to use the layers of muscle fascia in such a way as to close the defect where the bowel pushes through without causing undue strain on the suture lines causing the sutures to tear through, and thus making the repair fail. I learned how to put in a regional block and repair a groin hernia without either a general or spinal anesthesia, although it is a lot more difficult than just walking in after the anesthetist has the patient asleep for the repair. The advantage is this: after the repair is completed, it can be tested by having the patient cough and see that everything holds together.

An example would be Andrew K, an elderly man, who I operated on with a regional block. After the repair, I had him cough to test the suture lines, and then I walked him back to his room under his own power. One could not do this with a general anesthetic. Usually I used spinal anesthesia for my cases, since it was easier and a little more reliable, but it was nice to know how to do a regional in the event that the spinal didn't take completely.

There was another patient, Ted, a neat old guy, who worked around town mowing lawns and working as a handyman for odd jobs. He had developed a hernia that had enlarged to the size of a football as more and more of his intestines descended into his scrotum. He did not have any money to have it fixed, so I told him I would do it as a charity case. There were quite a few of those cases in the days before Medicaid or the "Great Society." The two problems with his repair were the long standing stretched tissues, and the problem of how to get all of his intestines back into his abdomen. Fortunately, with a lot of slow careful dissection of the adhesions, I was able to slide the bowel back through the dilated inguinal ring, gently close it, and make a few relaxing incisions so that I could pull the fascia together without undue strain. Ted was one of the happiest patients that I can remember, and one of the most grateful. He gave us a turkey for Thanksgiving. Unfortunately, he only got to enjoy his repair for about three years before he developed an inoperable lung cancer.

Today, with the various kinds of surgical mesh, the repairs have become much more simplified, and recurrences much less likely. We simply have to dissect out the hernia sac, tighten up the internal ring, cut our surgical mesh to the proper size to reinforce the weakened inguinal canal, and sew it in place. Someone is always inventing a better mousetrap.

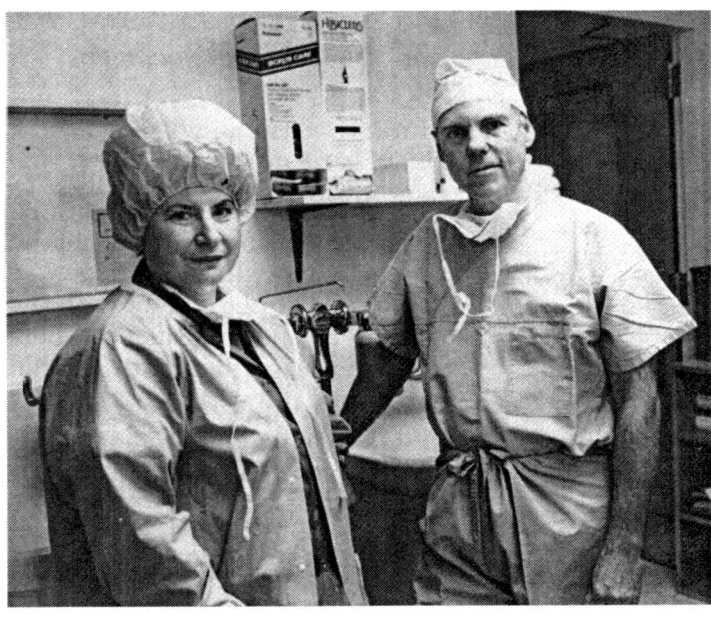

Scrubbing in with Lorraine Kuntz in 1989.

When we would get an abnormal Pap smear, we had to refer those cases to one of the Billings gynecologists for a procedure called colposcopy. A magnifying microscopic with a long focal length was used to look at the cervix under 60 power magnification and the doctor would try to identify the abnormality after painting the cervix with acetic acid to bring out the abnormality. Because there was usually a wait of several weeks before we could get them in for study, I decided to learn the procedure. There was a course being given at MD Anderson Cancer Hospital in Houston which was just what I needed. I enrolled in 1986, to learn the procedure. We had enough cases in Hardin that I could remain proficient in the technique. When I would locate the abnormal area by the acetic acid method, biopsies were taken, and frequently the cervix could be frozen to destroy the abnormal area. Acetic acid, when applied to the cervix, turns the abnormal area white in contrast to the normal areas, making it easy to define the borders. This added another dimension to our practice with fewer referrals to Billings. When we had a course given at our yearly Montana Academy of Family Practice meeting, I was able to help teach the course for those just learning the procedure.

When John March joined our practice, laparoscopic surgery was just beginning to be used and he had learned the procedures in his residency in California. We did a lot of tubal ligations, and although I had gotten good enough to do an open tubal through a keyhole incision just big enough to get my index finger into the abdomen and hook the tube to bring it up into the incision, a closed procedure was better since the patient didn't have to stay overnight in the hospital. The post-op discomfort was also much less. We ordered the special instruments and TV monitors with the tiny laparoscopic cameras, and now added another type of surgery that could be kept at our local hospital. We could also do the diagnostic exams for endometriosis and chronic pelvic pain that was a significant part of our gynecologic practice. Later, laparoscopic cholecystectomies became a part of our practice. This was a tremendous step forward in shortening hospital stays and reducing postoperative pain which resulted from the long subcostal incisions that were required for adequate exposure of the gallbladder. At that point, although I did most of the open cases, and those requiring exploration of the bile ducts, we decided that Dr. Ostahowski should be the one to become the expert at laparoscopic abdominal surgery, and as such, he did all of those cases.

Flexible scopes were being introduced in the 1980s, so we purchased one to do flexible sigmoidoscopies. This made the procedure a lot more comfortable for the patients. We could see twice as far as the old rigid scopes would allow us, and this made diagnosis of colon cancer more accurate. Most of the cancers would occur in the lower 25 cm. of the colon, but in the late 1990s the percentage began to change and colonoscopy of the entire colon became the gold standard. We sent Dr. Ostahowski to school again to be our physician for this procedure. He has become as skillful in this procedure as any of the gastroenterologists that I have seen.

With the advances in understanding stomach ulcers after we learned about helicobacter pylori and its close relationship to ulcers, gastroscopy was the next skill to learn. This involved looking into the stomach directly, instead of relying on X-rays to diagnosis ulcers. This now became the procedure of choice. I went to Billings on a number of occasions to observe the procedure on patients that I referred. There was a course offered in Orlando, Florida, for those who were already familiar with using flexible scopes, and Marlene and I traveled there in the spring of 1992. The hotel where the course was held was nice, and their dining room seemed above average, so I ordered the beef stroganoff for supper. About 4 hours later I paid the price with a devastating case of staph gastroenteritis. I spent the entire night in the bathroom with vomiting and diarrhea. When morning came, I was dehydrated and weak to the point of passing out when I stood up. If I had such a patient in my care, I would have hospitalized him for IV fluids, but I had flown a long way to take the course and I was not going to give up. Several times during the course of the lectures, I had to leave to lie down and try to sip some fluids and not throw them up. Fortunately, the syllabus had most of the lecture material in it, allowing me to read what I had missed. The next day was hands on with the gastroscope using models, and by that time I had rehydrated somewhat. The following day was test time and I passed with flying colors. We spent the next 2 days visiting Disney World and getting suckered into buying a time share, which we finally sold a few years later without ever having used it. Doctors are not the best businessmen!

When I arrived home, the hospital ordered a gastroscope and I soon had patients scheduled for the procedure.

When I finished my residency in 1961, I felt comfortable handling most situations that were presented to me, but medicine is constantly advancing and education never stops. We either keep moving forward by acquiring more knowledge and skills or we go backwards. Constant study, lots of reading, and continued medical education is a necessity for physicians, especially those in Family Practice.

CHAPTER 32
THE ACADEMY

In the early part of the twentieth century, general practitioners began to be looked upon as not being competent enough, and the specialists were beginning to be more of a force in medicine. The first specialty board was ophthalmology which became a reality in 1917, followed by otolaryngology and seventeen other specialty boards by 1940. Specialization was based on advanced education degrees, testing, and other requirements. General practitioners lost ground as they were progressively being prevented from more and more hospital activities and procedures. The numbers of general practitioners began to decrease in relation to the general population increase, and the AMA realized that this was becoming a problem. There still needed to be a doctor who could take care of the whole family and correlate their medical care. The American Academy of General Practice was established in 1947 in an attempt to encourage continued medical education, improve the image of the general practitioners, and forge them into a unified group to gain some political clout. With this, family medicine was reborn.

Residency programs were developed, providing three years of additional training to prepare these new doctors with the ability to care for the problems of the whole family. The term "Family Practitioner" was now being substituted for the term "general practitioner." The American Academy of General Practice had its name changed to the American Academy of Family Physicians in 1971, requiring doctors to maintain continued medical education and recertification every three years. The American Board of Family Practice was established in 1969, and in order to belong to this specialty board, a physician would have to complete an approved residency, pass a rather rigorous written exam, maintain continued CME, and be re-certified every seven years. This was even stricter than the other specialty Boards who did not require any re-certification.

I joined the AAGP shortly after finishing my residency and became board certified in 1969 when the board was established. I became President of the Montana Chapter of the Academy of Family Practice in 1973. However, the year before that, I was Vice President, and as such was in charge of the scientific meeting for that year. Most of our meetings were held in the northern part of the state, which made it hard for the doctors in eastern Montana to travel the long distances across the state. I decided to have the meeting in a more central place, and at first glance, Billings seemed to be the most logical place. Then a better idea came to mind, if I could pull it off.

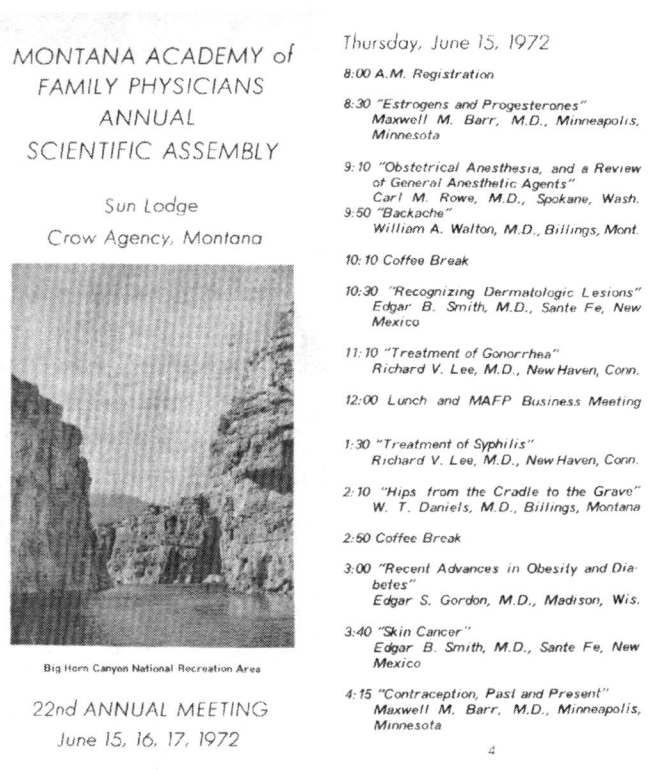

MONTANA ACADEMY of
FAMILY PHYSICIANS
ANNUAL
SCIENTIFIC ASSEMBLY

Sun Lodge
Crow Agency, Montana

Big Horn Canyon National Recreation Area

22nd ANNUAL MEETING
June 15, 16, 17, 1972

Thursday, June 15, 1972

8:00 A.M. Registration

8:30 "Estrogens and Progesterones"
Maxwell M. Barr, M.D., Minneapolis, Minnesota

9:10 "Obstetrical Anesthesia, and a Review of General Anesthetic Agents"
Carl M. Rowe, M.D., Spokane, Wash.
9:50 "Backache"
William A. Walton, M.D., Billings, Mont.

10:10 Coffee Break

10:30 "Recognizing Dermatologic Lesions"
Edgar B. Smith, M.D., Sante Fe, New Mexico

11:10 "Treatment of Gonorrhea"
Richard V. Lee, M.D., New Haven, Conn.

12:00 Lunch and MAFP Business Meeting

1:30 "Treatment of Syphilis"
Richard V. Lee, M.D., New Haven, Conn.

2:10 "Hips from the Cradle to the Grave"
W. T. Daniels, M.D., Billings, Montana

2:50 Coffee Break

3:00 "Recent Advances in Obesity and Diabetes"
Edgar S. Gordon, M.D., Madison, Wis.

3:40 "Skin Cancer"
Edgar B. Smith, M.D., Sante Fe, New Mexico

4:15 "Contraception, Past and Present"
Maxwell M. Barr, M.D., Minneapolis, Minnesota

4

A couple of pages from the meeting brochure.

The Sun Lodge, on the Crow reservation, had excellent facilities for a meeting, and a completely different perspective than we had experienced in the past. The problem was, as in many of their financial endeavors, Crow politics played a huge part in the success of their ventures. It had been open for about six years and then was closed because of financial mismanagement. It then reopened with Ramona Howe at the helm. Previous to that, she had been the manager and had operated it successfully for several years, but then had been fired due to tribal politics and a change of tribal administration. The tribe rehired her again and things were going okay, but I was still worried that by the time of the meeting things could again change and it would close, leaving me with a meeting, but no meeting place. I decided to run the risk, and started getting the meeting planned.

In addition to an excellent program of current topics relating to family practice, we had some really topnotch speakers to talk about these areas of medicine. There was one afternoon off from lectures for the doctors, and instead of golf or tennis, as was frequently the case, I planned boat rides on Yellowtail Lake and a barbecue for the doctors, with elk, moose, or deer, whatever their choice. Actually it was all beef with a few different spices added, but they never knew the difference.

We had a great meeting, everyone learned a lot of up-to-date information, and the doctors got exposed to a little Crow culture with a performance of Indian dancing at the evening banquet. I have to tell you, I sweated out those last few months prior to the meeting, and true to my expectations, the Sun Lodge closed again a few months later, never to open again. Oh well, all's well that ends well, as far as our yearly meeting was concerned!

CHAPTER 33
ADVANCES IN MEDICINE

Medicine has made huge advances in the last 150 years. How did we get here so fast? The short answer is "On the shoulders of giants." I have written about several of these milestones in the previous chapters, but now I am going to discuss what I consider the ten most important advances in that short span of years. There are many to choose from, but here are mine in chronological order. The ones I have previously covered will only be discussed briefly, but the history of some of the others are important enough to spend a little more time delving into their past.

Three really important advances, the discovery of ether and other anesthetic agents, followed by Lister's concept of antiseptic surgery, and later by Jenner's discovery that inoculation with cowpox could prevent smallpox, are topics that I previously covered. That said, I will begin with the discovery of insulin as number four on my list of ten.

Diabetes has been known to physicians for thousands of years, but was poorly understood. Doctors knew that the urine of diabetics was sweet, and it was known as the sugar disease. Diabetes was believed to be a digestive disease and physicians tried to modify diets to include more meat and fat in the diet, and restrict the sugars and starches. Inevitably, the patient became malnourished, dehydrated, acidotic, and then death occurred. Doctors suspected that the pancreas was involved with some mysterious digestive secretion, but could not isolate it. They removed the pancreases of normal dogs and noted that the dogs became diabetic. Grinding up the pancreas and making an extract was not successful, but occasionally the blood sugar of dogs was temporarily reduced. The extract was always too impure to be of any value. Researchers noted that there were islands of cells in the pancreas that looked different from the other glandular cells, and they also differed in that they had no ducts leading from them for any digestive fluids to drain. These were called the Islets of Langerhan after the doctor who first described them in 1869. These cells were thought to be the source of this mystery hormone that lowered blood sugar.

Enter Dr. Fredrick Banting. He was a young orthopedic surgeon who served in WWI as a Canadian medical officer. When he returned home to Toronto and opened a practice, business was slow. To supplement his income he took on a part time job teaching anatomy and physiology in the local medical school. On October 30, 1920, as he was preparing a lecture about the pancreas in the physiology class, he read an article about the relationship of the Islets of Langerhan to Diabetes. The author had described a case in which a large stone had formed in the main pancreatic duct and obstructed it. This caused a backup of the digestive juices and destruction and atrophy of the acinar or gland cells, but it left the islet cells intact.

Banting was thinking about this when he went to bed that night, and, unable to sleep, wrote himself perhaps the most important note that a sleepless person could ever write to himself. Ligate the pancreatic duct of the dog, wait six weeks for the pancreas to degenerate, and then remove the pancreas and attempt an extraction from the remaining islet cells. If the mysterious substance was in the islet cells, it would not have been destroyed by the now absent digestive enzymes.

He went to Dr. J.J. Macleod at the University of Toronto with the idea. After a cool reception by Dr. Macleod, who believed that Banting was too young and inexperienced to take on a project that other more learned scientists had failed, Macleod finally relented. He gave Banting a small lab with meager facilities and an assistant, who was a medical student named Charles Best.

Their work began on May 17, 1921. They ligated the main pancreatic duct of dogs, waited for the pancreas to atrophy, extracted the internal secretion, and then injected it into other dogs that had been made diabetic by removing their pancreases. The studies were positive and their blood sugars were reduced. This procedure was laborious and could not be used on a large scale. Now, with the help of Dr. Macleod and a biochemist, J.B. Collip, who was skilled in extracting the insulin with various concentrations of alcohol and acetone, they tried using fetal calf pancreases, which had a much larger number of islet cells.

When they finally got a sufficiently purified extract, they tested it on a 14 year old boy named Leonard Thompson. His blood sugar tests dropped dramatically and his sugar excretion in the urine also was significantly reduced. Acetone bodies, a result of excessive fat metabolism, were also reduced as the boy was now able to metabolize glucose.

I could go on for pages about all of the jealousy, infighting, mistrust, and animosity that went on among these four discoverers of insulin, but somehow they rose above it, and the Nobel Prize was given to Banting and Macleod in 1922. They acknowledged Best and Collip by sharing the prize with them. The production of insulin required a large facility for the sudden request by diabetics all over the world, and the job was ultimately given to the Eli Lilly Company. Finally, diabetics did not have to die at an early age from lack of insulin. The downside of this, however, was that they could now live long enough to pass on this genetic defect to their children.

Banting's life came to an untimely end on February 20, 1921, when a plane in which he was the only passenger, developed engine failure and crashed as it was returning to base. Despite all of the controversy about who should have gotten the most credit for the discovery of insulin, it has saved the lives of millions of people throughout the world, and has been a huge milestone in the advancement of medicine.

Number five on my list would have to be aspirin. The time line of this drug goes back to 1500 B.C. when it was recorded that the Egyptians used dried myrtle leaves containing salicylic acid to treat back pain. Hippocrates, the father of medicine, used Willow bark, which also contained salicylic acid, to reduce fever and treat mild pain in 200 B.C. The salicylic acid was made commercially in 1874 but was too irritating to the stomach, so an attempt was made to make an ester or a salt which would be better tolerated. Charles Gerhardt was the first to synthesize ASA, or acetylsalicylic acid, but he had some problems and did not pursue it further.

It was not until 1897 that Felix Hoffman, a chemist at the Friedrich Bayer Co. was able to synthesize it by reacting acetic anhydride and salicylic acid. According to legend, Hoffman gave this product to his father who suffered from arthritis and could not tolerate salicylic acid. He obtained good relief, but the mechanism of action was not really understood until much later. As is usually the case, there was a great deal of arguing about who was the first to discover how to make aspirin, and there were several patent infringement suits argued in the courts. Since Bayer could not stop all of the competitors from producing aspirin, the trademark was finally genericized in 1921.

And now, I need to explain a little about how aspirin works, and some of its good and bad effects. It probably has had the most wide spread use of any drug ever used. It was recognized early on that it could reduce fever, and relieve a wide variety of minor pain conditions. Its use in arthritis was widespread and when I started in practice, it was really the only drug that we had for rheumatoid arthritis. We used huge doses, averaging about 16 of the 325 mg. tablets a day. If there was ringing in the ears, we cut back by one or two tablets a day until it stopped. Interestingly, I never noted much gastric irritation reported or significant bleeding until we started asking about it and checking for intestinal bleeding much later in my practice. Rheumatic fever was quite common when I was in medical school, and aspirin was part of the treatment to prevent heart valve damage and the joint inflammation that was part of the acute process. Aspirin works by inhibiting substances called Cox-1 and Cox-2 prostaglandin enzymes which cause the damage to the joints. Later, it was found to inhibit platelet activity and to be of great help in treating heart attacks and stroke. There are a number of cancers that may receive some benefit from the use of aspirin also. Premenstrual syndrome and migraine headaches are also benefited by aspirin.

The most serious side effect from aspirin, although rare, is Reyes syndrome. After certain virus diseases, especially Chicken Pox, aspirin can induce this condition, which carries a 35% mortality. The cause of death is usually liver necrosis. Children should not be given aspirin due to this rare side effect. Bleeding, gastric irritation, and ringing in the ears are also side effects that should be looked for. Aspirin can also cause hemolytic anemia and severe allergic reactions in some patients. It may also aggravate asthma in some children.

All side effects considered, aspirin still remains one of our most important and successful drug. The number of heart attacks and strokes that it may have prevented or modified are legion, and its effect on certain cancers are still being investigated. Long live the Bayer Company!

Number six on my list is cortisone. In order to talk about this subject, I should review a little about endocrinology and the adrenal glands. These two little caps sitting on top of the kidneys were little understood in early medicine. Dr. Thomas Addison, a British physician, first described a condition from patients who had died from a fatal wasting illness, and he noted that their adrenal glands had wasted away or degenerated. Since nothing was know of their function, he decided to investigate this problem. The condition is now known as Addison's Disease.

Thomas Addison received his doctor of medicine in 1815. He was very interested in skin diseases, and he described the particular bronze pigmentation in the disease named for him. He showed in numerous autopsy specimens the relationship of the bronze pigmentation and the atrophied adrenals. He noted the other symptoms of weakness, fatigue, sweating, headache, weight loss, and salt depletion that accompanied this ultimately fatal illness. Later it was found that extracts of beef adrenals could treat the condition, and it was felt that these unknown compounds were required to control multiple bodily functions.

In 1930, Dr. Edward Kendall isolated six compounds from the adrenals. Later, in 1941, Dr. Philip Hench, a rheumatologist at the Mayo Clinic, noted that after certain stressful situations, the arthritis in many patients improved. He surmised that a hormone secreted by the adrenal glands was responsible for their temporary improvement. In 1948, one of Dr. Kendall's compounds, cortisol, was tried in a patient and the results were astounding. The inflammation, swelling, and pain were dramatically reduced and the patient could become ambulatory again. One observer commented that these patients improved to the point that they could now walk from their beds to the autopsy table. Both Kendall and Hench received the Nobel Prize for their contribution in the discovery and investigation of cortisone.

The expense of synthesizing cortisone kept it from being widely used since it was made from ox bile, thus a better way had to be discovered. This leads us to Dr. Percy Julian, the grandson of a slave in Alabama.

Percy Julian was born in1899, and grew up in Montgomery, Alabama. There was only limited education for blacks, but he managed to get through high school and he entered DePauw University and graduated as class valedictorian. When he initially left for college, he was seen off by his grandfather, who, as a slave, had two fingers cut off as punishment for trying to learn to read and write. Percy Julian got his Ph.D. from the University of Vienna in 1931, but was unable to get a professorship since these opportunities were very limited for blacks. After he went to work for the Glidden Paint Co. as a research chemist, he synthesized a number of important drugs and compounds from soybean protein. He discovered that he could use a wild sweet potato from Guatemala, the Yam, to synthesize cortisone, thus reducing this prohibitively expensive drug to just pennies a gram. He was truly one of the giants of chemistry during his lifetime.

Cortisone could now be used in a wide variety of inflammatory conditions. Both rheumatoid and osteoarthritis responded dramatically to small doses. A number of serious inflammatory conditions could now be treated. Asthma and allergic reactions, in addition to severe skin diseases were now treatable. Ulcerative colitis was brought under control, as was polymyalgia rheumatica. Almost all the connective tissue and autoimmune diseases could now be influenced by one of the cortisone derivatives. As the middle of the nineteenth century unfolded, we were now able to get a better handle on how to treat a number of previously untreatable diseases. Our march toward conquering disease was speeding up!

The "crazy" people have always been hard to deal with. By that, I mean the delusional, the manics, the psychotics, schizophrenics, and those having delirium reactions. In the more distant past they were locked away, placed in straitjackets, or otherwise confined so that they would neither be a threat to society, or to themselves. Sedation with opium, alcohol, barbiturates, bromides, or paraldehyde was sometimes used, but none of this was satisfactory. And so we come to my seventh milestone, the development of antipsychotic drugs.

In 1937 the antihistamines were discovered, and one class, the phenothiazines, was of interest to a French surgeon, Henri Laborit in 1949. He was using them as an aid to anesthesia. They seemed to produce a calm state, and he thought that they could also be used in psychiatry for the more agitated patients. In January 1952, he persuaded a psychiatric colleague to try out one of the variations called 4560RP, which was ultimately named chlorpromazine. They gave it to a 24 year old man with mania, who then became calm and manageable. Several trials were then begun at St. Ann Hospital in Paris, and 38 psychotic patients were injected with between 75 and 150 mg. of chlorpromazine daily with very good results. The wards of mentally ill unmanageable patients could now be controlled, and the nurses and staff of these hospitals could now better interact with their patients. This new drug was spoken of as the psychic penicillin.

Dr. Kinross-Wright, a psychiatrist at my medical school, Baylor, was very active in investigating chlorpromazine, or Thorazine, which was its brand name. As medical students, we were able to observe the dramatic change in behavior of the schizophrenics, who, before the medication, were actively hallucinating and hearing voices. They could now be better reached with psychiatric intervention. The voices would stop and the delusional behavior could be controlled. The "last resort" treatments of electric shock and "insulin coma" were now a thing of the past as far as schizophrenia was concerned, although ECT (electroconvulsive therapy) is still used in some cases of severe depression. Great numbers of mentally ill patients were released from the mental hospitals all over the world, and were able to be managed with outpatient treatment as long as they remained on their medication. There were side effects from long term use of these drugs, including tremor and sometimes permanent twitching, but it was a small price to pay for the dramatic change in these patients' lives. Later, second generation antipsycotics with fewer side effects and even better control of symptoms were developed.

Depression was always a serious psychiatric condition, and was usually treated with counseling, and psychoanalysis of the patient's problems. Occasionally, electroshock treatments were given for the most resistant cases. Lithium salts were found to be helpful for the manic depressive cases as early as 1948. It is interesting to note that Dr. Robert Cloud established a hospital, the Lithia Springs Sanitarium, in 1890, for treatment of addiction and compulsive behavior. The natural waters from the springs were high in lithium, fluoride, potassium, and calcium, which probably accounted for the beneficial effect. With improvement in understanding brain chemistry- especially the metabolism of serotonin, dopamine, and epinephrine- the tricyclics and then the SSRI's, or selective serotonin reuptake inhibitors, were developed. These made it much easier to treat depression through a combination of drugs and counseling.

Finally, the anxiety disorders were able to be better treated with drugs other than sedatives such as barbiturates. Meprobamate, better known as Miltown, was discovered and put on the market in 1955. Everyone wanted to be on this drug after a hard day's work at the office. It was heavily advertised to the doctors and used excessively until it was found that it had addictive properties. It fell out of favor with the discovery of Valium, one of the family of benzodiazapams. This drug has stood the test of time for anxieties, in addition to its use in surgery, and even for treatment of acute seizures.

We seem to be a society who want a quick fix for the consequences of our stress filled lives and fast life styles, with either legal prescription drugs, or illicit ones bought on the street corner. We need to work out other methods to relieve our stress other than drugs. Exercise, involvement in community projects, relaxation techniques, taking long walks, and playing with our animals would go a long way in making our lives fulfilling enough so that mind altering substances should not be needed.

The discovery of polio vaccine gets my vote for number eight in the war on disease and suffering. Polio was one of the most feared conditions that parents worried about for their children each spring and summer. I remember my parents worrying each year if one of my friends, or, heaven forbid, if I would be a victim of this terrible affliction. As you remember, one of my closest friends, Dr. Herb Schaumburg did come down with it, and was left partially paralyzed. There would be no more going out for long passes, or playing catch with the softball any more with him.

The first major polio outbreak reported in the United States occurred in Vermont in 1894, with 132 cases reported. In 1916, over 9,000 cases were reported in New York City alone. In 1921, Franklin D. Roosevelt contracted polio, leaving him with significant paralysis in the lower extremities. The iron lung was developed in 1928 to assist respirations during the critical early phases of the disease. There were large epidemics of polio following WWII with more than 20,000 cases reported each year, and in 1952, there were 52,000 cases reported.

Jonas Salk, the developer of the first successful vaccine, was first working at NYU on an influenza vaccine for the military, during WWII. He then moved to the University of Pittsburgh in 1947. He began a relationship with the National Foundation for Infantile Paralysis, and he began to work on a vaccine for polio. After eight long years of research, he developed a killed virus vaccine which produced antibodies that protected against the disease. In 1955, over two million school children were inoculated with the vaccine. I got my three shots along with my classmates during the 1957 school year at Baylor.

Dr. Albert Sabin, the researcher who developed the live virus vaccine, came to the United States from Poland as a fifteen year old immigrant youth. He had to learn English in school, but was a good student and he also participated in several after school activities. He received his medical degree in 1931, and he became interested in polio research. He was able to show that polio virus not only grew in nerve tissue, but could also live in the small intestine. This was very important since the live virus vaccine that he later developed could stop polio from living or multiplying there, unlike the killed virus of Jonas Salk. He found that there were a large number of people in primitive countries who had antibodies against polio but who had never had the disease. He found three strains of these weakened viruses and further attenuated them to use as the basis for his vaccine. The ease of a live virus that could be given orally made it especially good for mass immunizations throughout the world, where less skilled health workers could give it.

With the use of these two forms of polio immunization, we have almost accomplished what we were able to do with smallpox, in reducing a devastating disease to a rarity. The Salk vaccine was given in a mass immunization in 1957, and polio cases dropped dramatically. The Sabin vaccine became available for mass use in 1962, and I remember the campaign that we had here in Hardin, immunizing everyone with the five drops of vaccine on a sugar cube. Our turnout was huge, and it was very rewarding to see so many people show up for their "treat."

Birth control gets my vote for number nine on the ten most important advances in my 150 year time frame, since in days long past, childbirth was a risky business. Women died from infection, hemorrhage, malposition of the fetus, or sometimes they just "wore out" from too many pregnancies

Pregnancy and conception were not well understood, until Leeuwenhoek, with his microscope, showed the tiny sperm moving in the seminal fluid, which gave the medical community some vague idea of what conception was all about.

Egyptian camel herders found that if they inserted a large pebble into their camel's uterus, the camel would not get pregnant on the long caravan journeys and thus was born the first IUD. In 200 A.D. a Greek physician, Soranus, suggested that using a mixture of tobacco juice, ginger, olive oil, and pomegranate pulp inserted into the vagina would prevent pregnancy. I can think of a more esoteric reason why it would, if you get what I mean. Another remedy that seems a little more logical to me was a small sponge soaked in vinegar or lemon juice. Condoms made of animal intestines and membranes were used in the middle ages, but were more for prevention of syphilis than for prevention of pregnancy. You may remember Charles Goodyear for making tires, but in 1884, his rubber vulcanization process made possible the development of rubber condoms, and his company produced millions of them.

As we began to understand more about contraception and birth control, Congress, in 1873, passed the Comstock law that made it illegal for physicians to distribute birth control information or devices through the mail. This was due to pressure from religious groups. Physicians circumvented the law by calling them feminine hygiene products. Margaret Sanger, the first women's health advocate, saw her mother die essentially of exhaustion after 18 pregnancies and 11 live births. She established the American birth control league and disseminated birth control information in spite of the Comstock laws. In 1916 she opened the first family planning clinic. She teamed up with Katherine McCormick, a philanthropist, and they helped fund research by Gregory Pincus, who was studying hormonal biology. In conjunction with Frank Colton, a chemist at the G.D. Searle Company, they developed a pill, Enovid, for gynecologic disorders, which eventually became the first birth control pill. Because of strict birth control laws in 1957, Searle was hesitant to market it as an oral contraceptive, but after FDA approval in 1960, this finally occurred. In 1965 the Supreme Court case of Griswold vs. Conneticut overturned the Comstock law and legalized birth control for married couples.

Although Searle monopolized the market for awhile, many pharmaceutical companies got into the act, and it was found that the amount of estrogen and progesterone in the original Enovid was much larger than was needed. With the smaller dosages, side effects were much less, with still virtually 100% protection from pregnancy. Taking a page from the camel herder's book, IUDs were developed and these have become the contraceptive of choice throughout the world with the exception of the USA. Progesterone inserts put under the skin were very popular for awhile, and I can remember scheduling one or two patients a day for a long time for this procedure. They were good for at least three years before they had to be removed and new ones inserted. With the advent of laparoscopic surgery, done as an outpatient, tubal ligation remains the best long term solution for many women. We have come far in becoming masters of our own destiny.

Number ten on the list brings up a larger number of options, all of which could fit by someone's standards. I chose the heart-lung machine and open heart surgery as my number ten choice because I was there in medical school when it was happening. Dr. Debakey and Dr. Cooley were in the forefront of this technology, and as medical students, we were there working up those patients for this cutting edge surgery. We were able to be in surgery observing the procedures as they were going on.

All of the congenital heart defects, septal defects (holes in the heart), and valve problems could not be corrected in a beating heart. A machine was needed to divert the blood around the heart, and oxygenate the brain and body so the heart could be stopped, opened, and repaired. Cooling the brain, heart, and body also gave extra time to do the repairs. Also, the pump should not damage the blood cells either, in the course of its pumping action. One of my classmates, Sam Luce, whom I wrote about earlier, decided to try to make one to mimic or do the current heart lung machines one better. My other classmate, Julie Martin, and later to be Julie Martin-Luce, had connections at the Hughes Tool company where her father was an engineer. He agreed to take Sam's plans and present them to the engineers. They constructed a pump with a roller to push the blood forward, similar to how the pumping of the atrium and the ventricle work. The blood was then run through an oxygenator and returned to the body. When it was finished, it was a small compact unit, unlike the massive devices currently in use. He gave it to the medical school which used it successfully in the dog lab for some of their research, but it never seemed to make it for use in humans. It does show, however, that someone pretty far down on the food chain can still come up with innovations and good ideas.

Before the heart lung machine was developed, most of these young children were relegated to life as invalids until they died from heart failure. The numerous cases of mitral stenosis could sometimes be temporarily helped by a procedure in which the right atrium had a purse string suture placed in it, and then a cut made in order to slip the surgeon's finger in with a small knife blade attached. He would then cut the constricted valve by feel to open it up enough to allow more blood flow through and help correct the back up that caused the lungs to fill up. After the heart lung machine was developed, the heart could be stopped, opened, and the valve totally replaced with either a pig valve or a mechanical valve of several types. The aortic valve could also be replaced and the septal defects could be repaired to prevent mingling of oxygenated and un-oxygenated blood across the two sides of the heart. As medical students, we got quite good at listening to the heart sounds, and diagnosing the multiple varieties of defects that could be present. Currently, an echocardiogram will give a 3-D moving picture of the heart function and valve function so that nothing is left to chance. Today, young physicians may have lost this skill in diagnosing the abnormalities with the stethoscope alone, but such is the road of progress.

Well, there you have them, my ten most important advances of the last 150 years. There are certainly a lot more that could qualify, but one has to start and stop somewhere, and these give a fairly good picture of medicine's remarkable progress that I have been privileged to see and be a part of.

CHAPTER 34
MY GREAT ADVENTURE

Everyone needs at least one "great adventure" in their lives. Mine was a trip as the doctor to accompany my friend, Dr. Elwyn Simons, on his yearly archeological dig in the desert sands southeast of Cairo, Egypt. Elwyn is director of the Primate (Lemur) Center at Duke University and has a special interest in early mammal fossils of the Eocene and Oligocene eras. Each year, through a special arrangement with the Egyptian government, he is able to take a team of graduate students and paleontologists to excavate several sites for fossils in the northern desert of Egypt. These are shared with the Geological Museum in Maadi. I was invited to join the group, and with much anticipation I accepted the invitation. What fun it would be to rub elbows with all those scholars, and in addition, learn how to retrieve the fossilized bones with a dental pick and a paint brush. We would also get to visit a lot of the ruins in that area that tourists don't get a chance to see.

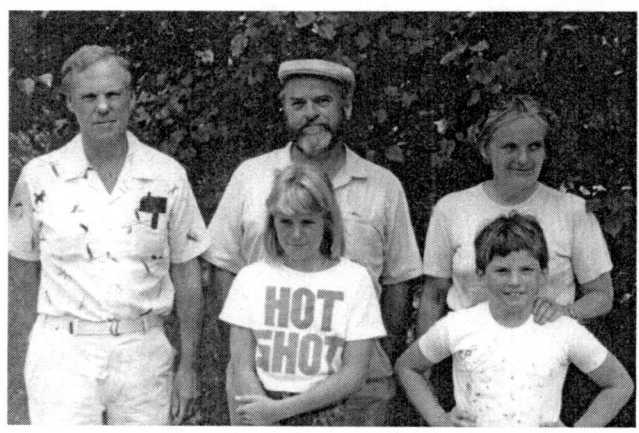

With Elwyn Simons and his family.

I began making preparations for the trip which was to be in October 1991. In addition to my passport, I also needed a visa and a desert permit for the trip. I thought that I should also learn a little Arabic before hand, so I purchase the Berlitz Arabic for travelers. I packed my bedroll, a compact suitcase, and a good sized "fanny pack" that housed some dried fruit, nuts, peanut butter, deer jerky, two small cans of chicken, candy, matches, and a Swiss Army Knife. Bandaids, Kleenex, a compass, string, and a few other assorted items filled the rest of the compartments. I wanted to be sure that I had a small supply of food, in the event that it wasn't available in an emergency. Some medical supplies and antibiotics were packed in my suitcase. I was finally ready for the trip. I would fly from Billings, Montana, to Denver, and then catch another plane to New York. There I would meet up with the Duke team at the JFK airport. We would then fly to Cairo via Rome, spend one night in a small hostel, and then head out into the desert in SUVs.

Well, things don't always go as planned, as the story will soon indicate. I was scheduled to leave on October 10, 1991, with the first leg of my journey on Northwest Airlines at 7:00 A.M. The night before had been very busy, and I was called back at 1:00 A.M. to take care of a patient who was hemorrhaging from a miscarriage. I had to perform an emergency D&C on her to get control of the bleeding and get her stabilized. I finally got back to bed about an hour later. Somehow the alarm got turned off, and I awoke, wondering what time it was. In October it was still dark until about 7 A.M. I turned on the light and the clock said 5:55 A.M. The airport in Billings was 48 miles away and the plane was scheduled to take off in an hour. Marlene and I jumped out of the bed as if it was on fire and dressed in seconds. My bags were all packed by the front door, so we were on our way in just over five minutes. We did break a few speed limit laws on the way to Billings, but the highway was essentially deserted at that time of the morning. I jumped out of the car with all my gear flailing about me and raced up to the ticket counter. I asked the attendant if I was too late, and she pointed to a plane already in the air and answered in the affirmative.

I felt pretty disappointed about the situation, so I asked when the next flight was scheduled. She said the next flight that connected all the way to Cairo would not be for about a week. Boy, was I down! I decided to call our travel agent, Jim Court, who had "saved our bacon" before on another vacation. Jim looked at all the schedules and found that there was another flight on Continental leaving at 9:00A.M. that went through Minneapolis, with a plane change, and then on to New York. The rub was that it went to La Guardia airport instead of JFK. That would require an inter-airport bus shuttle to get me to JFK, all requiring additional time. Jim said that I should present my Northwest ticket to Continental and explain my hard luck story to them. Maybe they would take my ticket without my having to buy an additional one. If my connections didn't work out, he said, "Just enjoy a weekend in New York and come home."

I went to the Continental desk to plead my case, and to my surprise, they accepted my ticket and got me on the 9:00 A.M. flight to Minneapolis. That flight was on time, but I was already two hours behind. There was also a one hour layover before their flight to La Guardia which made it an almost impossible situation. When I arrived in Minneapolis, I noticed the gate next to my arrival gate had a sign indicating it was a flight to La Guardia that had been delayed thirty minutes and was now preparing to leave. I asked the attendant if I could get on that flight, and she told me that since there were vacant seats, it would be no problem. I got on, they closed the doors, and we took off. That lucky event had caught up my lost time, but I would end up at another airport, where I would again lose time.

The plane landed at La Guardia on time, and I rushed off the plane with my bedroll, suitcase, and fanny pack bouncing up and down. I asked an attendant the direction to the inter-airport shuttle and was directed to an escalator on the first level. I found that they were on a one hour schedule and the shuttle had its door open, and was ready to leave. "Wait," I cried out and the attendant looked up as he was closing the door. I was on it in a flash! The trip took about thirty minutes, but I was picking up time with each leg of the journey. I arrived at JFK, went through the appropriate gates, and my goal was in sight. The plane to Rome didn't leave for thirty minutes. I found Elwyn and his group, who were a "sight for sore eyes." I said, "Have I got a story to tell you!" Soon we were on our way to Rome. They had not issued me a confirmed seat on the next leg and that worried me a little, but I was on a roll.

I had been studying my Berlitz book of Arabic to learn a few simple phrases, and as luck would have it, a lady of mid-east appearance was seated next to me with a small baby. Here was a chance to practice my Arabic. So, in my finest accent, I said, "tifi gae**mīl**," which translates as baby pretty. She thanked me with the word "**shok**ran," which means thank you. I began to think later that if I had pronounced the word pretty with the accent on the first syllable, it would have been "**gae**mael", or camel, and I would have said, "Your baby looks like a camel." That would not have been a very good way to start a conversation.

It was a long flight and we all had to bed down for the night as best we could. Finally, we arrived in Rome and deplaned. I was trying to make sure that I had an assigned seat, but the attendant said the computer was down but not to worry. That still didn't help since there was another man who didn't have an assigned seat and he was getting irate and loud. They told him if he didn't quiet down they would call security. It was time to begin boarding and still I hadn't been given a seat assignment. By now, I was getting a little panicky. Finally, as most of our team was boarding, they called my name and gave me my seat number. What a relief it was for me, but I do not think that the other man got aboard, even though he had a confirmed reservation.

We landed in Cairo, and Elwyn started negotiating with some cab drivers to get the gear and supplies for the expedition into the city. Getting a cab at the right price is quite an accomplishment since all the cab drivers were competing with each other, yet trying to make the most profit that they could for the trip. Finally we arrived at our hostel and checked in. We were required to give up our passports which were taken to the local police station and held as long as we were in the city. This bothered me a lot, since, with government bureaucracy, who knew if they would disappear, especially since we were not given a receipt for them. We drove to a small restaurant and had an interesting meal of tasty Egyptian cuisine, followed by a few beers and some interesting discussion of the deteriorating infrastructure in Cairo since Britain's exit from the country.

We were up early the next morning for a tour of Cairo by our guide and leader, Dr. Simons. After driving around the streets and observing some of the homes and museums, we headed to Giza to visit the pyramids and the Sphinx. Giza is six miles southwest from Cairo.

The three pyramids are known as the Pyramids of Giza, although there are a number of smaller ones close by. The largest of these three was the Pyramid of Cheops, built by Khufu. It rose to a height of 1,450 feet, and initially was 1,481 feet tall. The other two pyramids were Chaphren and Mycerinus. The giant stone blocks of the Pyramid of Cheops are exposed as stairs stepping upward, because some stones and facing of better quality limestone were taken away to become parts of medieval buildings in Cairo long ago. Some of this polished limestone was also used by some of the later pharaohs to enhance their own pyramids. With some difficulty we climbed up the pyramid for a better view of the surrounding area. It was quite a sight. These three pyramids were built by the rulers of the fourth dynasty.

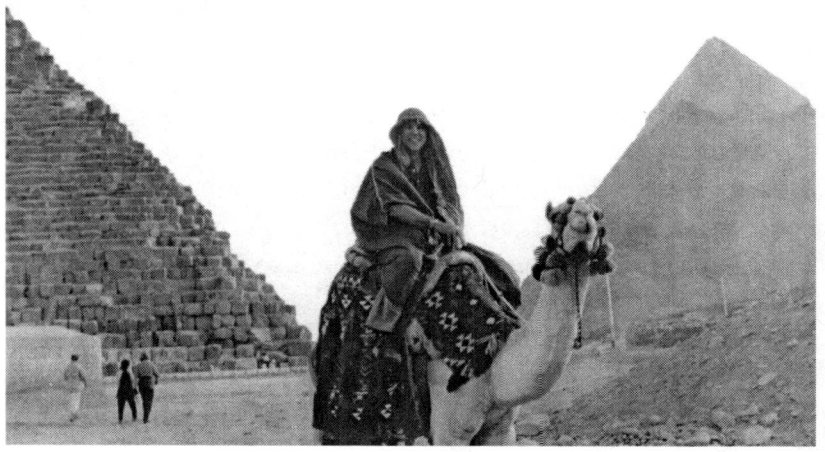

My first camel ride in front of the Pyramids of Giza.

One could get a good view of the Sphinx from there, so naturally that was our next site to visit. The basic facts about its origin are still debated, and much has been written in this regard. Some think it represents the likeness of King Khafre, who is credited by some as the builder not only of the Sphinx but also of the second pyramid. This would date it from about 2520 B.C. to 2494 B.C. Some historians date its origin as much earlier than the time of Khafre and claim that he only uncovered it from the burial sands of time. A theory put forth by a French scholar and reinforced by several others noted that water erosion dated it to a much earlier time when the region was much wetter and floods from the Nile were greater. This would date the inception of the Sphinx to about 1,500 years before the beginning of Egyptian civilization, and most scholars find this impossible to believe since they have not found any evidence of an advanced civilization that early.

The missing nose of the Sphinx is also a point of debate. One legend is that it was destroyed by a cannon ball from Napoleon's soldiers. This is probably false, since sketches made by a Frederick Norton in 1737 showed the Sphinx without a nose before Napoleon's soldiers arrived in Egypt. There also was a beard at one time which has fallen off. It is stored in the British Museum and has never been reattached. Some felt that it may have been added at a much later date than the original construction. That concluded our tour, so we headed back to the hostel and began packing our gear for the trip into the desert. We collected our passports and were on our way.

We noted that sanitation was not the best in Cairo, and the infrastructure had deteriorated considerably since the British moved out after WWII. We passed a large garbage dump on our way out of town, and the garbage was not buried, just left in large piles, with hoards of flies buzzing around. In the desert there were no roads, and one sand dune looked just like the next, but our drivers knew exactly how to get to our camp, which was about twenty miles from Cairo. The sand was hard packed and the tires did not sink into the sand unless the crust was broken for some reason. Then, one could get mired in the soft underlying sand. Finally, we arrived at camp where a number of tents were set up with metal and canvas cots for our bedrolls. There was a larger cooking tent where we all ate, and where our Egyptian cook prepared the meals. There were several latrines which were just deep holes, dug into the sand, surrounded by some canvas barriers for privacy. The nights started warm, but as the night progressed, the temperature would drop, and by morning I had my bedroll zipped up. After 7:00 A.M. breakfast, we would get into the SUVs and head out to the dig sites. We each carried our quart bottle of water wherever we went, in the event of some emergency or breakdown. At noon we would head back to camp, eat, and have a brief rest in our tents. Then we would head out for more fossil collection until just before sunset, when we would return for supper. All of the specimens were carefully wrapped in toilet paper to prevent breakage. After supper they were unwrapped, identified, and then again wrapped and cataloged. Discussions of politics, social issues, and a little study of Arabic followed, over a few bottles of Stella beer until bedtime. We found a few large scorpions around the cook tent, and captured them in a large glass jar. There were always a few moths attracted to our lanterns and they provided food for the scorpions. It is interesting to note that spiders usually suck their prey dry, but scorpions entirely consume their victims, so the next morning, there would be no trace of the moths that we put in the jar the night before.

I learned the knack of finding the small fossilized bones and then carefully exposing them with the dental pick and brush. There were a lot of fossilized fish bones that we came across, but they were not important finds. Once I found something that I could not identify and I asked Elwyn just what I had uncovered. Much to my chagrin, he told me that it was fossilized crocodile dung. I saved it, thinking it would make an excellent conversation piece.

I did a little exploring away from camp, always being careful to get my bearing from some landmark when I went over a dune and out of sight of the camp. Elwyn took me to one area where there was a hillside of broken pottery jars. He said these were left from the days when Heroditus, the historian, traveled with the Roman Legion through the area thousands of years ago. I collected a few fragments for souvenirs. What history lies in those shifting sands! Once, on the way back from digging, we visited a partly buried temple in a place called **Dime**. We had lunch in the shade of some of the partly sand filled rooms. Several of the columns were still standing and there were broken pottery jars again on the hillside. There were a few fragments of beautiful blue tiles called **Faiance** that had been fused onto a clay base and probably were gorgeous blue walls adorning the temple thousands of years ago. How they could create these layers that long ago is beyond me.

There were no significant medical problems for me to deal with except for a few sprains, a case of sunburn, and a few minor bowel problems. Interestingly, there was no traveler's diarrhea, even though we were eating fresh salads and some uncooked vegetables. Finally, it was time for me to leave the expedition and do a little individual sightseeing. I was driven into town where I purchased a ticket to Luxor and the Valley of the Kings. I spent the night at the same hostel that we used the first night and the next morning took a cab to the airport and was on my way for more exploration.

When I arrived in Luxor, I caught a cab into town and headed to the hotel Luxor, where I stayed during my time there. My cab driver made a deal with me to pick me up the next morning and drive me to some of the interesting sites and act as a tour guide. That afternoon I walked to the Tourist Bazaar and did a little shopping. I found a beautifully carved silver bracelet with gemstones that I wanted to get for Marlene. The shopkeeper wanted more than I wanted to pay, so I tried to leave twice, and each time the price got lower. Finally, with crocodile tears in his eyes he sold it to me for about thirty dollars, American. I think we were both satisfied.

Next, I found a store that had some small perfume bottles as their specialty. I found a number of them to purchase; and, if there had been room in my suitcase, I could probably have been a middle man for a lot of merchandise. I was ready to pay the owner, but he said that we would have to have refreshments first. I haven't had a store owner treat me that special before. He brought out Egyptian coffee and served it in small cups. It was so strong that my spoon could have stood up in the middle without support, but it was quite good. There was a pasta buffet at the hotel that night, so that was where I ate supper. Breakfast the next morning was coffee and several kinds of very good bread. There was some left over in the basket so I wrapped that up and put it in my fanny pack to enhance my tube of peanut butter for lunch.

My guide was on time and we went into the bar for a cup of tea and to get acquainted. He had a lot of questions about America. Misconceptions can frequently place a wedge between people of different cultures. I have two good examples as evidence.

During our visit he said, "Can I ask you a question about your religion? Is it true that you Christians actually eat flesh and drink blood during your worship?" That took a little explaining for him to understand that the bread and wine of Communion was only symbolic of Christ's body and blood that was shed for us to atone for our sins. False impressions can easily arise from incomplete knowledge. I remember another time when Marlene and I were visiting our son Craig when he was stationed in Germany. We visited an old walled city, Rothenburg, and had a young woman tour guide who took us on a sightseeing tour around the city in a horse drawn cart. When we got to a corner tower of the wall she said, "That tower is haunted by a ghost." She didn't know much more about it, but when I looked at a brochure, it all became clear. She was a black girl from Morocco and was obviously Muslim. Knowing very little about Christianity, the fact that the tower was known as the "Tower of the Holy Ghost" meant nothing more to her than there was a ghost up there. Again, incomplete knowledge can lead to some pretty strange conclusions.

My taxi driver was a chain smoker and when I told him about the health hazards, he said, "I know, but life is hard, and cigarettes get me through it." He told me that his brother was lying at home with probable appendicitis, but since he didn't have the money, he couldn't be seen by a doctor. I was tempted to go see him myself.

My tour took me to the temple complex of Karnak which is about two miles northeast of Luxor. It was an interesting morning. Most of the columns and walls were covered with hieroglyphics, and were somewhat worn by the elements over time. This brings up the interesting story of the discovery of the Rosetta stone, which was the key to unlocking this dead language.

The ability to read and understand the ancient hieroglyphics was lost about 1400 years ago. The Egyptians were dominated by the Persians until Alexander the Great defeated them and brought his army to Egypt. He was welcomed by the Egyptians and almost considered a God. After his death, Egypt was ruled by Ptolemy 1, his son, and then by a series of successive Ptolemies until Ptolemy V. This Ptolomy had a series of decrees inscribed on stone tablets in several languages and placed before a number of temples. These consisted of procedures, canceling certain taxes, forgiveness of certain debts and a number of other acts and rules. During the succeeding years, Egyptian and Greek languages were used simultaneously, followed by Latin when the Romans controlled Egypt. Within one hundred years, all knowledge of the written hieroglyphic language was lost. All of this immense knowledge was essentially left untapped until 1799.

Napoleon's soldiers captured an area in the Nile Delta, and one of the soldiers was using some of the stones as building blocks to reinforce a fort. He found a stone of black basalt with inscriptions in three distinct languages, with part of the top containing some hieroglyphics broken off. The middle group of symbols was an Egyptian script called Demotic (a type of abbreviated hieroglyphic text), and the third set of inscriptions was Greek text which he recognized. He took this stone to a group of scholars there in the town of Rosetta, and they recognized it to be a royal decree of Ptolemy V. Silvestr deSacy was the first to decipher the symbols that composed the words Ptolemy and Alexander. Additional symbols were added by several other linguists, and in 1802, Stephen Weston translated the ancient Greek on the stone. Thomas Young determined that people's names had to include several hieroglyphics grouped together and then encircled to form a cartouche.

Then came Jean-Francois Champollion. He was a master linguist. He began his study of the stone in 1808. He read all that was previously written about it, and finally published his results in 1822. He determined that some hieroglyphics were pictures that represented a concept, and some were phonetic sounds. Others enclosed in a cartouche represented a Pharaoh's name. From that point, he was able to decipher this dead language and unlock the hidden mysteries of the past.

I spent some time in Karnak's temple and then returned to my hotel. I took a boat across the Nile to the Valley of the Kings and bought tickets to visit several of the tombs. After I had seen several of the tombs it was time for a little lunch, so I raided my fanny pack for some of the bread that I had saved from breakfast, along with my peanut butter tube. I opened a small can of chicken that I had saved. As I was starting to eat, I noticed several very emaciated dogs, with their ribs showing, looking longingly at my lunch. Well, that did it! I would go hungry, and they would get my lunch and whatever else I had left in my fanny pack including my deer jerky and some cheese that I was hoarding. At least, for a day, they would have a little something in their empty stomachs.

The following day I decided to walk from my hotel to the temple of Luxor, which was about half a mile from my hotel. There were numerous donkey drawn carts on the street and all of the drivers were calling out to take me for a ride for a few Egyptian pounds. I finally grew tired of saying no thank you or just ignoring them, so finally I decided to pretend that I could not understand English. When the next driver came by, in my best accent I said, "Ich verstehe sie nicht." (I don't understand you). He replied in even better German, "Fahren Sie mit mir, mein Herr. Es ist sehr billig." (Ride with me sir, it is very cheap). So much for that tactic! I walked along the Avenue of the Sphinxes and then into the temple. There were many small tour groups scattered around, so I found one where the history was being given in English, and listened to the lecture before moving on to other areas of the temple. It was very impressive and there was so much to see in such a limited time. I would be wasting words to try to describe the grandeur and enormity of those structures. It needs to be seen to be appreciated. Several days of sight seeing and it was time to catch the plane back to Cairo.

When I arrived, I caught a cab back to the same hostel. I told my cab driver that I would be catching an early flight to the airport the next morning. He pleaded with me to let him take me back to the airport again. I think that he slept in the lobby that night in order not to miss the fare. I gave him a generous tip, (bakshish), and our trip was uneventful. When I arrived in Rome, there was a baggage handler's strike and the flight to New York was delayed several hours, so naturally my connection from New York to Denver had to wait until the next day. Finally I was home, with my ancient pottery fragments, my piece of blue tile, some fossilized crocodile poop, my perfume bottles, and a lot of great memories.

CHAPTER 35
THE CHANGE

Throughout the previous chapters, I have hopefully covered the first part of my book title, which was the bedside part of the book. Now it is time to move forward to the last part of the title, the HMO, and see how we got here. When I started in private practice, there was very limited medical insurance, and certainly no safety net to fall back on except the county welfare system. Of course, when I started in practice, office calls were four dollars and the cost of a tonsillectomy was fifty dollars. If a patient was really destitute and on welfare assistance, the county did authorize some medical payment. Shortly after I arrived in Hardin, I made an arrangement with the county to provide anything that I felt capable of handling for $450.00 a month for all of the indigent patients in the county. This included office calls, hospitalizations, surgery, and deliveries. There were no reports to file, no lists of patients seen, and no bills to submit. If I couldn't handle the problem, the patient was sent to Billings for more involved treatment at the county's expense. That was the ultimate example of a no paperwork arrangement.

Nurses were given free care, as were all of the clergy. I think that the dentists and their families were given a 50% discount also. It's a wonder I made any money at all. If a patient was not indigent enough for the county's criteria, but really needed medical care, it was given on a pay me when you can basis. Sometimes there was a little bartering involved for things like elective surgery. I remember having a fence painted, and a brick planter made as compensation for a hysterectomy. Once we got a buffalo roast from a patient. My uncle once told me,

"If you go to Montana, you're going to be paid in chickens and eggs." He was partly right!

Slowly, the price for medical care began to rise, but I always tried to keep mine under the Billings fees. Medical insurance began to be more popular as time went on, and Blue Shield and Blue Cross were two of the major players in the state. Doctors had to join the plans in order to participate and be paid directly by them. They did have to agree to follow the fee schedule, however. The doctors were not regulated by anyone else except their peers, their hospital medical boards, and the State Board of Medical Examiners.

In 1965, all that changed. John Kennedy has previously said in his famous speech, "Ask not what your Country can do for you, but what you can do for your Country." Then Lyndon Johnson became president and essentially said, "What can your Country do for you?" The "Great Society" was born.

I really didn't spend much time thinking about all the things that were going on at that time, since I was so involved with patient care. In looking back now, there were many things that needed fixing, and Lyndon Johnson had plans to fix them all. He had been given a mandate by the people by virtue of an overwhelming majority in both the House and the Senate, so he was able to enact sweeping changes in the way our country viewed society with little opposition. Before I review the changes relating to medicine, I think I should comment on the way he envisioned the government's responsibility toward the people.

He saw government as providing a "hand up" rather than a "hand out" to that segment of our society that was impoverished by a variety of reasons. Education was a cornerstone of his program, and through a series of loans, scholarships, and grants, he saw to it that anyone with the necessary brains and ambition could go to college. He established Head Start which enabled those children coming from deprived homes to have enriching social and educational experiences so they could better compete with those children from well-to-do families. The school breakfast program was begun which fed those thousands of children that went to school on empty stomachs. The food stamp program helped feed more than 8 million households.

Lyndon Johnson saw his Great Society's mission as one in which poverty would be eliminated and racial injustice brought to a halt. Segregation in housing, buses, accommodations, toilets, and water fountains were eliminated by the 1964 Civil Rights Act. If you remember, Marlene had not been exposed to the problem, coming from Montana. She really didn't know what to make of it all when she moved to Houston in 1957 during my senior year, and saw the "Colored" water fountain in Foley's department store.

Social Security benefits were dramatically raised, which lifted 12 million elderly above the poverty line for the first time. Nursing home benefits were also established, making it possible for many elderly to receive care which was previously provided only by their families. The Office of Economic Opportunity launched 12 programs covering every facet of society. These included legal services, migrant education and health clinics, Job Corps, Vista, Head Start, Senior Citizens Centers, Community Health Centers, Foster Grandparents, and Upward Bound, among others.

I remember seeing a cartoon of two hippies walking down the street, and in the caption under the cartoon one was saying, "What should we do today?" The other replied, "First, let's go down and collect our welfare checks, then pick up our food stamps, stop by the free VD clinic, check on our subsidized housing, and then we can go down and protest in front of the local draft board." Many people thought the government had gone too far in its desire to provide for everyone. Truly, many did take advantage of the situation. There was a lot of fraud, graft, and cheating that went on, as would be expected when suddenly the candy counter was left unattended. All of these programs required huge outlays of money by the federal government, and the escalation of hostilities in Vietnam was also costing a lot of money.

Medicaid was created July 30, 1965, through Title XIX of the Social Security Act. Each state administered its own version, but there was matching money to all of the states. Benefits did vary from state to state, and some people actually moved to the states with the highest welfare and medical benefits. It took only a few months to establish residence, and thus eligibility. It turned out that Medicaid was much more expensive than was calculated, as were most government programs. The states were over budget, and soon it was apparent that cuts would have to be made. Many expensive procedures such as bone marrow transplants for children were just not covered by many of the states. The alternative was either to let your child die, or move to one of the few states that covered it and establish residency there. Hospital inpatient days had to be cut, so much of the elective surgery was changed to same day admission. This made patients a little inconvenienced by having to be at the hospital sometimes as early as 5:00 A.M. in order to be ready for 7:00 A.M. surgery, but it actually worked out fairly well, and did affect significant cost cutting. Several surgeries that previously had been kept overnight before being dismissed were made outpatient procedures, and these patients had to be dismissed before midnight.

It became necessary to establish codes for every conceivable procedure performed by doctors so that appropriate payment could be determined and paid accordingly. Procedure payments were significantly reduced from the doctors' usual and customary charges. Hospital length of stays for all patients was determined by the diagnosis code. If a patient had, say pneumonia, and exceeded the length of stay, the doctor would have to write a request for additional days or the hospital and he could not continue to charge for services.

Since there were drastic reductions in what doctors were allowed to charge, many stopped accepting Medicaid patients, or at least stopped accepting new patients. One way to increase reimbursement, however, was to use the procedure codes to advantage. Many doctors, or at least their coding staff, learned to play the procedure book like a musical instrument. For instance, if the doctor was doing an exam of the ear as part of a regular visit, and there was wax obscuring the view of the ear drum, he would either clean it out with an ear curette or wash it out. There is a procedure code associated with this and an additional charge could legitimately be made. Before all this procedure coding, we would just clean out the ear at no charge and continue with the exam. Likewise, in a geriatric visit, I would always examine the feet, check pulses and examine skin integrity. If the toenails were long and needed to be trimmed, I would take a few minutes to do it at no charge. There is, however, a surgical procedure code for this, and podiatrists make a living doing this as part of their profession. Another inequity in charges in the dermatology area was in treating lesions such as warts or premalignant actinic keratoses by freezing. It takes only a few minutes more to freeze a dozen than to freeze just one. There is a code for freezing one, and then a second code with a lesser fee for the next ten and so forth. Before coding was in effect, I would just charge for a freezing procedure, but with the reduction in payment mandated by Medicaid, use of the code book enabled one to make up for it, and one could run up a rather exorbitant charge. Also, the type of visit was a bone of contention. They were grouped into focused, expanded, detailed, and comprehensive. I will discuss this later in the chapter. The list of ways to enhance reimbursement goes on by how innovative a coder can be.

Medicare was also enacted in 1965, with part A covering hospital costs. A deduction was taken out of the social security to cover that cost. Part B was optional for physician, outpatient care, emergency room, ambulance and some more ancillary services, but most people paid the premium for part B to have these services, and the premium was also taken out of their social security check. Eighty percent of the cost was covered for these services, as was the case for part A, so most people bought insurance for the 20% not covered. There was a deductible also. Naturally, the federal government recognized that they could not pay usual and customary fees, so these were reduced significantly for both the physician, hospital, and other providers. As is usual with most government programs, they underestimated the cost of the program, and further fee reductions were enacted, and increased deductions from social security payments were made.

In order to correlate payment for service received, medical visits were classified as focused covering one system or complaint, expanded covering 2-4 systems, detailed covering 5-7 systems, and comprehensive covering 8 or more systems. Examination of these bodily systems had to be documented in the doctor's notes in order to justify payment, and audits were conducted to make sure that no fraud was present. More rules and regulations continued to be required, making the time factor for a medical visit more about paper work and documentation, and less about hands on medicine. This is what usually happens in many government programs when good things are carried to extremes.

Another example of this is the confidentiality law that protects information of patients from being given out to unauthorized personnel. Obviously, that is a good thing, but the law now contains thousands of pages, covering every conceivable situation, with severe penalties for infractions. Lab reports cannot be given to spouses for convenience sake; prescriptions can't be picked up by unauthorized relatives; conversations have to closely guarded so that they cannot be overheard; screens had to be installed on clinic and hospital computers so that a passerby could not see the screen as he or she walked by; inpatient rosters could no longer be posted in hospitals for the benefit of visitors; and, a whole host of other rules, too numerous to document, were put in place. When I was gathering information for this book, it was extremely difficult to have access to patients' charts from 40 years ago, even though they were records written and signed by me. The patients were deceased as were the people authorized to give me the permission to view them, so it was a Catch 22 situation, with the records inaccessible.

There are large numbers of uninsured people in this great country of ours, and there is a ground swell of talk about how to handle this problem. Obviously, we need to do something, for it is unthinkable that a rich country such as ours with the best medicine in the world cannot care for its moderately poor. So say some, but is it really true? These patients do not have a regular physician because doctor's visits are too costly, and these patients do not have an advocate for reduced fees, such as Medicaid, Medicare, and private insurance companies. A focused visit for something as simple as an earache costs about $62, but if the physician dares to put his stethoscope on the chest or examines any other part of the patient, it changes to an expanded visit for $85. Most patients would think the doctor was not very thorough if he stopped at the ear. Now, if the patient has an advocate, such as the above entities, the maximum fee is set at a much lower rate, namely $34 for a focused visit or $55 for an expanded one. Many of these non-insured patients do not have a regular primary care physician, and use the ER for their services. They don't need an appointment for this, and they just go in and are seen, but the rub is that it is incredibly expensive. An average ER visit is probably in the range of $450, and an ER visit for a simple laceration, about $650. I can remember when the charges were $25 for the facility charge and $15 to sew up the laceration. If any lab or X-rays are done, then the price really increases, and most people presenting to the ER do need some diagnostic tests. Patients can plead inability to pay, and most hospitals have funds set aside for charity or reduced payments if the patient qualifies. This does require proof, such as an income tax return or some sort of documentation.

The Hill Burton Act was passed in 1946, which provided funds to build and renovate hospitals in medically needy areas. There were strings attached, however, one of which was to provide an appropriate amount of charity care for 20 years. This was later amended to "in perpetuity." Our local hospital received these funds and gave charity care as a yearly percentage of the grant for 20 years until it was written off. Continued charity care then continued as a slightly lower percentage of revenues collected. They don't advertise for people to seek free care, however, and indigents have to be smart enough to request it.

Because medical costs were rising so rapidly, companies that provided health coverage for their employees were feeling the pinch and looked for ways to reduce their costs. As a result, Health Maintenance Organizations (HMOs) were developed. There are several types, some with salaried physicians who act as gatekeepers and who have to be seen first before referral to a specialist can be made. HMOs monitor their physicians to make sure that they are not giving too much or too little care, and are not costing the HMO too much with too many expensive studies or high priced brand name prescriptions instead of generics. Capitation is usually part of the package, which means that a national average of costs for a patient of a certain age is figured into the premium and if the HMO can stay under that value, they make money. If not, they lose. The practitioners are encouraged to keep this in mind when dispensing service.

Physicians or other primary care providers such as nurse practitioners or physician assistants are assigned a tight schedule and pushed to see as many patients as possible. Visiting about the kids and how one's golf game is going is not part of the conversation. The numbers of specialist's referrals are closely monitored. Some insurance groups will give patients a policy limiting them to just the doctors on their roster, who have agreed to accept lower fees. Frequently, choice of hospital is also limited. This agreement will result in a lower premium, since the insurance company has negotiated a lower payout to the providers. The name of the game, however, is really rationing of care.

Kaiser Permanente is an example of a very successful HMO. It began in California but also has an extensive network in a least five other states. My friend, Dr. Jim Miech, who started out with me after our residency eventually ended up there. He retired from practice after working for them for twenty years, with a nice pension. He had nothing but good things to say about their system and the working conditions. His experience was certainly not like some of the others that I described above, but not all hospitals, clinics, or businesses for that matter, are equally successful.

There are two other large groups of people who receive medical care provided by the government: namely, the Indian Health Service and the Veterans Administration. I was an Indian Health Service physician and served my military obligation in that capacity. There are approximately 2,000,000 Indians, or more politically correct, Native Americans, in this country, and through their treaties with the government, they are guaranteed free medical care as long as they live on the reservation. In Montana, there are seven reservations, the Flathead, Blackfoot, Crow, Cheyenne, Ft. Belnap, Ft. Peck, and Rocky Boy, comprising more than 67,000 Native Americans who live on these reservations. There are also many more Native Americans who live off the reservations in surrounding communities. Many have Medicaid cards, especially those living off the reservation, and thus have dual access to care, either through private physicians, or by returning to the clinics or Indian hospitals set up to care for them. Medicaid is their primary source, however, and the Indian Health Service is permitted to bill Medicaid for services that they render in order to supplement their own budget. The same goes for Medicare and private insurance.

The Veterans Administration also provides a significant amount of medical care which is government sponsored. In 1907, there were 7.8

million veterans enrolled in the program and 5.5 million treated. The Veterans Health Care Eligibility Reform Act of 1996 provides a two tiered system. Category 1 provides medical care for those veterans with service connected disabilities of 50% or more, disabilities incurred in the line of duty but not yet rated, disabilities related to Agent Orange, and certain radiation type conditions. Also included in Category 1 are veterans with limited incomes or elderly veterans. Category 2 includes all other veterans, and a means test is applied with some fairly complicated rules to determine eligibility. Co-payments are usually required both for inpatient and outpatient services. Any insurance coverage that the veteran has is billed to the insurance company by the VA for reimbursement. There are a number of other benefits such as limited free transportation to and from a VA facility, reduced costs for prescriptions, medical screening, immunizations, and several other perks. If I went into too much more detail, your eyes would probably begin to glaze over, so we'll leave it at that.

So where do we go from here? Undoubtedly, our country will be looking at some type of universal health care system in the future. We need some type of coverage that won't bankrupt the small employer, the individual, or, Heaven forbid, the country. Before I go much further, a few comments from some great writers are in order. Mark Twain once said, "Suppose you were an idiot. And suppose you were a member of Congress.... But then I repeat myself." George Bernard Shaw said, "A government which robs Peter to pay Paul can always depend on the support of Paul." Ronald Reagan said, "The government is like a baby's alimentary canal, with a happy appetite at one end and no responsibility at the other." Finally, P.J. O'Rourk said, "If you think health care is expensive now, wait until you see what it costs when it's free!" Every program that the government runs, if one looks at past history, has been inefficient, over regulated, underestimated, and dotted with fraud and corruption. The crooks always seem to find a way to tap into the system and steal from it. Private insurance coverage seems to work better in the long run, since they do have a bottom line, unlike the government. It may turn out that even Medicaid and Medicare would be better served by letting private insurers handle the job.

225

When one speaks of "Universal Health Care" he needs to define what it means. Is this a right, a responsibility, or a privilege? I do not believe the politicians or health care providers even know what they are talking about. The "pie" is only so big and when we add hundreds of thousands of people to the mix, we will have to talk about that "dirty" word, rationing. Does that mean that for every life saving procedure that we add, we will have to subtract a non-lifesaving procedure? If we cover bone marrow transplants to save a child, do we tell elderly people with a cataract that since they can still see out of one eye, if they want it fixed then they have to pay for it out of pocket? Does it mean that for every liver transplant to save someone's life that we include, a hip replacement which is non-lifesaving will be an elective procedure and would have to be paid out of pocket by the person needing it? The list goes on and on. This will be one of the most complicated and difficult problems that our Congress will have to deal with in the coming months or years. The ramifications, when I start to think about them, give me a headache. The rules that we come up with will be unpopular to one group or another and "someone's ox will be gored" in the process.

Increasing health care to the large number of uninsured will require that we somehow cut the benefits that we will allow or control the costs. Cutting the benefits does not address the cause of rising costs. We are bogged down with forms for patients to sign, irrelevant questions that have to be asked in order to comply with protocol, and far too many expensive tests that we seem to need in order to either satisfy the patient's request or our need to protect ourselves from malpractice. This cuts our efficiency and the number of patients that we can see in a day. Right now, our annual health care costs are 16% of our GDP (gross domestic product) and exceeds two trillion dollars. We pay twice what other countries pay for health care that have better health outcomes. We are 19th among 19 developed countries in mortality that could have been benefited from better health care. American physicians, although presumably well paid, are the most unhappy in the entire world.

When we start changing how we deliver health care, I hope that we don't change this service too much in our quest to provide more than we are able to do at a reasonable cost. When service is "free," there are fewer restraints on the doctors to order expensive studies that are

226

borderline necessary in an attempt to "cover all the bases." There will also be more expectations from patients to have more done than is required, because it is "free." Believe me, I have already seen this time and again, and it will escalate. This will lead to more regulation and control, so that there may be committees to decide what tests one can or can't have, if carried to the extreme.

We had this situation a number of years ago when the MRI machines were just coming into use. They were expensive, and a state committee was formed to decide just how many units would be allowed in the state. It was decided that two would be enough, one in Billings and one in Great Falls. All other requests would be denied. There were all sorts of other regulations regarding numbers of nursing homes, numbers of beds, and a whole host of other issues that were taken up by this committee. As society's views changed, these restrictions in regulating medicine either just disappeared, or due to legal challenges, were withdrawn. Now, Billings alone has three MRI centers with a total of six MRI machines.

I do not envy the physicians and politicians who will have to make these decisions in the coming year or two, for it is a crooked road filled with potholes along the way, and our applecart could easily be upset without careful planning and fiscal responsibility to light the path ahead.

EPILOGUE

Well, there you have it, the story of a high school boy who had a chance encounter with the right person, at the right time, which brought a completely different direction to his life. If I had walked out to Westheimer Street five minutes later and missed that ride home, what would have been the effect both on my life, and all the lives that I have touched during the last fifty years? Life is full of event changing moments for all of us, but I still have that question in the back of my mind, "What if?"

It has been an interesting life, full of challenges, successes, obstacles to overcome, and many mountains to climb. The life of a physician is a difficult one, since one has to try to balance the needs of his family with the needs of his patients, which never stop, especially in a small town. Not all families survive this constant tug of war for the physician's attention. There has to be a lot of family support and understanding when the physician is called away from birthdays, graduation ceremonies, Christmas programs, band concerts, and a whole host of other activities important to the family, but interrupted by the constant emergencies that happen in a small town. Somehow, our family lived through it, and came out whole. I have to give thanks again to my wife and our three children, Lois, Marc, and Craig for their constant support and love, which brought us all through those early years when I was alone as the only physician. Finally, the Hardin Clinic became a stable group of doctors with Gary Ostahowski, Carol Greimann, and me as the core, sharing emergency calls and responsibilities.

And so the story that began over fifty years ago in Yellowstone Park draws to a close. I have carried the torch of medicine high for those many years and now have turned it over to those who come after. I say to them, "Carry it proudly," and in the somewhat modified words of J.F. Kennedy, "Ask not what medicine can do for you, but what you can do for medicine."

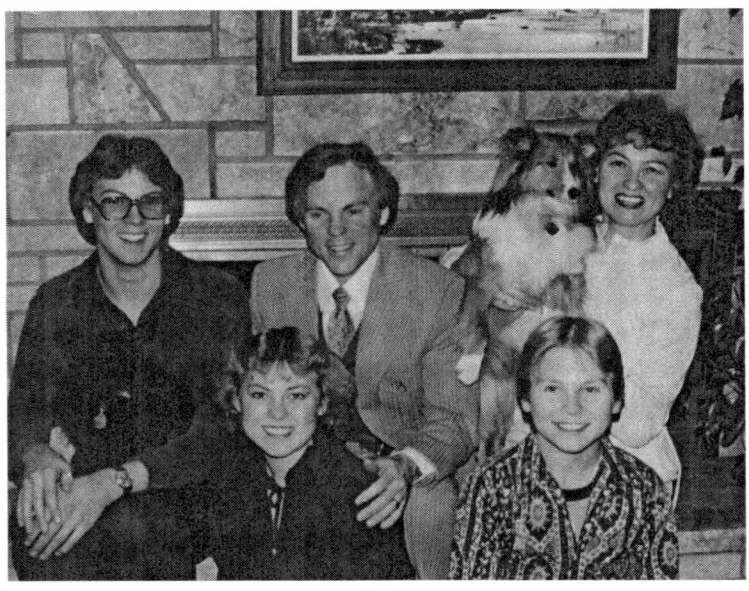

Our family growing up, Marc, Lois, myself, Craig and Marlene.

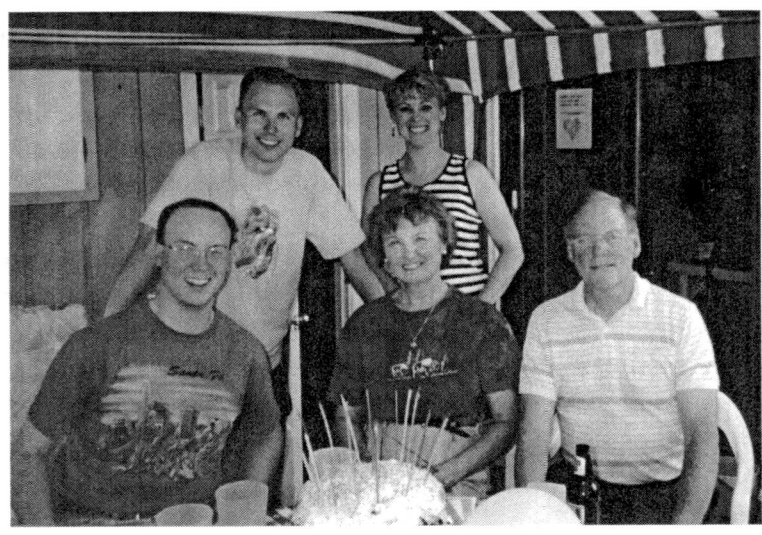

Our family all grown up. Marc, Craig, Lois, Marlene and myself.

I wrote a poem to Marlene on our second anniversary about how we met in Yellowstone Park, and I think now is the time to finish up that story and the book with a few more verses added to the poem.

'Tis fifty years since first we met,
In Yellowstone that day.
I courted you, I married you,
And skies turned blue from gray.

Of all the girls I'd known before,
You stood out from the rest,
And fifty years of marriage proved,
You surely passed the test.

Our children, three, were born and loved.
They grew up straight and strong.
We taught them of the ways of life,
And showed them right from wrong.

So life moves on to golden years,
The marriage vows do say,
And after fifty years of bliss
I love you more each day.

THE END

Printed in the United States
141159LV00004B/2/P

9 781440 123771